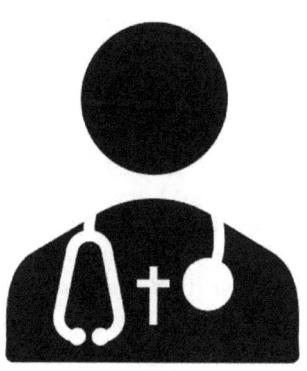

Pressed but not Crushed

Encouragement for Christian Junior Doctors

Published in partnership with:

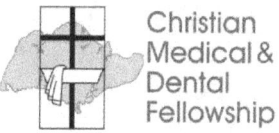

Christian Medical & Dental Fellowship

Pressed but Not Crushed: Encouragement for Christian Junior Doctors
Copyright © 2024 Hao Yi Tan

All rights reserved. No part of this publication may be reproduced, stored in a retrieval system, or transmitted, in any form or by any means, electronic, mechanical, photocopying, recording or otherwise, without the prior written permission of the authors, except in the case of brief quotations embodied in
critical articles and reviews.

Published in partnership with Christian Medical & Dental Fellowship (Singapore)
420 North Bridge Road,
#05-07, North Bridge Centre
Singapore 188727
Email: admin@cmdf.org.sg
CMDF Student Ministry: cmdfstudentminstry@gmail.com
Website: cmdf.org.sg

Produced by Graceworks Private Limited

All Scripture quotations, unless otherwise noted, are taken the Holy Bible, New International Version®. NIV®. Copyright © 1973, 1978, 1984, 2011 by International Bible Society. Used by permission of Zondervan. All rights reserved.

eBook ISBN: 978-981-18-9821-1
Paperback ISBN: 978-981-18-8893-9

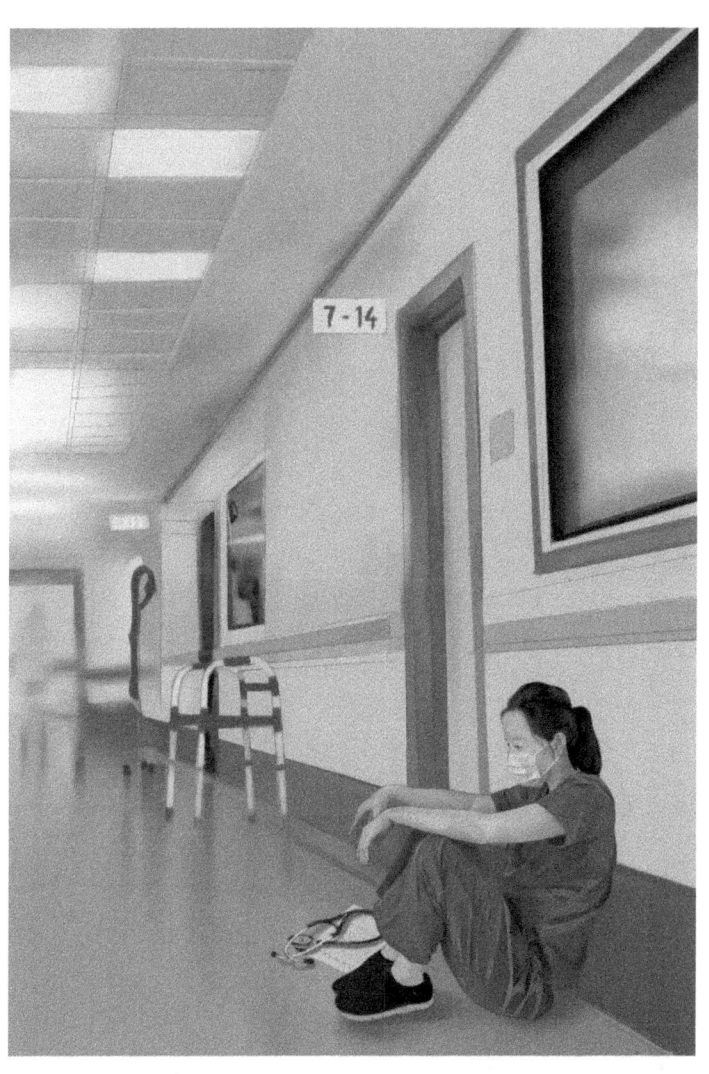

ARTWORK BY DR REGINA TAN

CONTENTS

Foreword by Dr Goh Wei Leong 1

Introduction 5

PART 1: THEOLOGY OF WORK 13
Why do we work? – God's Design and Redemption of Work 15

What do we really worship? – Idolatry and Idleness 33

PART 2: WORK AND OUR LIVES 55
Work-Life-Faith Balance 57

The Junior Doctor and the Church 68

Direction and calling in Medicine 76

PART 3: CHALLENGES AT WORK 83
When we look at our Patients – Attitudes of Christian Doctors 85

When we make mistakes – our response to medical errors 93

When we Fail – Dealing with Defeat 106

When we become Cynical – Negativity in our hearts 122

PART 4: MENTAL HEALTH AND WORK 133
Mental Health and Burnout 135

Anxious for nothing 161

Depression 173

Epilogue: Hope in the Lord 189

FOREWORD BY DR GOH WEI LEONG

Two years ago, I was catching up with a junior doctor I meet from time to time. Some way into the conversation, he revealed, almost as a confession, that he was taking an examination to prepare to move to New Zealand. The combined demands of church, family, and work were suffocating him, he said. He felt exhausted all the time and was beginning to think that the only way to find the Holy Grail—the ever-elusive work-life balance—was to relocate to the promised land for overworked medical professionals somewhere down under.

A familiar tale? For this young doctor, and for many other young healthcare workers, work, church, and family have become an unending, mutually reinforcing cycle of sleepless nights and exhaustion. It would be too glib to dismiss this as an isolated case of a junior medic being unable to handle the demands of the local system. All of us know this chronic overwork, fatigue, and resulting cynicism is a systemic problem.

How do we, then, as a Christian community, help ourselves look out for one another? How do we help seniors in mentoring and providing genuine spiritual friendships to juniors—friendships that are not about giving well-meaning, perhaps unsolicited advice, but about holding spaces for younger doctors to rest without guilt and just have someone be there for them?

We are often told as Christians that the greatest command is to love one another as Christ first loved us, but how often does this exist on the level of the abstract? When we concretise this command, we must acknowledge that loving one another takes on different dimensions in the workplace. What we need is practical wisdom and handles (not necessarily solutions!). And this is what this book may provide for us.

Perhaps it is helpful to think of this little publication as chaplaincy in a book. Hao Yi, one of the co-authors, is a younger doctor that I have journeyed alongside in recent years, and he is one in the trenches with you. Nigel, another co-author of this book, is slightly older, and knows the challenges of medical practice well. They know intimately the truth that within our community who care for bodies and minds, there exists a deep need for the care of our souls. The other co-author of this book, Soo Inn, has for the longest time since relocating back to Singapore, been the chaplain of Singapore's Christian Medical & Dental Fellowship (CMDF). It seems fitting, therefore, that his passion for being present with our bone-tired healthcare workers has translated into this book-as-chaplain project, such that we may all carry care with us as we go about our workdays.

Many of us who have taken up this profession of healing are wounded, especially as juniors fresh out of medical or dental school. Working as junior doctors can deal us the wound of isolation of work, and it seems that the more patients one meets through the depersonalised structure of institutions, the lonelier we become. Perhaps we may feel stripped of agency, that the profession is no longer liberating, that we are not expressing the skills we've learnt, that the skills serve almost to increase your loneliness, that we are forced into a godless, mindless productivity measured by KPIs.

Perhaps we may feel that modern medicine does not help us to be better healers—or Christians.

In Henri Nouwen's beautiful book, *The Wounded Healer*, he exhorts the believer to "[make] one's own wounds a source of healing" (Nouwen, 2013, p. 88). We all, healers or otherwise, share the same wounds of our human brokenness. Yet, taken together with the shared hope we all have in Christ, we may yet be able to find healing in our sharing of these unresolved wounds. We hold our wounds up to one another in community, and together hold these wounds up to God, who empowers us to see more lovingly into ourselves and others as only Christ can. Is there anything more astounding than the fact that our Saviour uses broken people to heal one another?

This little labour of love, therefore, serves as an invitation to healthcare workers to consider how our wounds themselves can become a source of healing. Perhaps this book is a space where stories and people can meet—one in which we may yet find, in beautifully broken community, a path to be pressed but not crushed.

Many of us have experienced hospital corridors as spaces of apprehension, anxiety, or even horror. Perhaps, as we hold each other's wounds in community, there is a way that these hospital corridors will breathe life again. Perhaps there is a way from corridors of exhaustion and cynicism to corridors of life.

May we yet find this way together.

Dr Goh Wei Leong

International Christian Medical and Dental Association (ICMDA) Southeast Asia Regional Secretary

INTRODUCTION

Many junior doctors fresh out of medical school make the transition into working life every single year; a great number of us junior doctors find it a struggle due to a myriad of reasons. More importantly, however, many start to fall away from God in this transition, leaving churches and cell groups, and sometimes even walking away from the faith. The attrition rate is shocking and is at times even discouraging to those who have yet to make that transition. At the same time, however, it is almost universally expected that this will happen.

The most passionate of Christian medical students can be reduced to disgruntled and disillusioned doctors who seem to have lost our fire or worse—our faith. Christian doctors at the workplace struggle with many things all at once: workload, physical exhaustion, lack of time, lack of spiritual support, emotionally challenging situations, steep learning curves, and the list goes on. It would seem almost implausible to expect someone in their 20s to make this entry into the workplace unscathed, with their Christian faith unaffected by the harsh reality of work.

Pressed but not crushed

Sometimes, people assume that doctors are indestructible or immune to burnout, illness, or exhaustion. Some of us work and act like this is really the case! But the reality is that we (like all other humans) are weak, imperfect, and fragile. The Bible makes it crystal clear that without God, we are nothing. Paul writes in 2 Corinthians 4:7–10:

But we have this treasure in jars of clay to show that this all-surpassing power is from God and not from us. We are hard pressed on every side, but not crushed; perplexed, but not in despair, persecuted, but not abandoned; struck down but not destroyed. We always carry around in our body the death of Jesus, so that the life of Jesus may also be revealed in our body.

Clay jars are common household items, fragile and unimpressive. Paul's meaning here is that we as humans are these ordinary jars of clay, but we carry the gospel with us. The good news of the gospel is the most valuable treasure on earth. But this treasure and this all-surpassing power is not from ourselves; it is from God. This clear juxtaposition in imagery emphasizes God's great goodness and humility in including us fragile vessels in His mission to bless the world. This should make clear that our ability to bear this treasure is not from our innate beauty, strength, or intellect. It is in His great mercy that we are invited to partake in this ministry and be blessed as we do so. Additionally, it is important to consider *why* we are called to carry around this treasure in our fragile bodies. Verse 10 concludes that we carry this gospel with us so that Jesus may be revealed! Jesus is not just our source of strength to carry out this mission, but also the motivation behind it—He is the reason why we work in the first place.

For the Christian junior doctors, we find ourselves in an often stressful and profoundly difficult environment. At least for the time being, while we remain in the medical field, we are called to serve God through this profession and to give our best every single day. We are called to use our fragile and finite bodies (the clay jars) to carry the good news of Jesus (the treasure) to all those around us every day, blessing our patients and our co-workers both physically and spiritually. We are called to carry our cross daily and go wherever He calls us to, carrying this love of God and perpetuating it as He has commanded us to do.

As God's children who work in medicine, we will inevitably be found in difficult positions as we work out our calling. We will be stressed, and we will go through trials of many kinds. Yet, God protects and comforts His Children, even as we are sometimes called to do His work in places that are frighteningly exhausting and seemingly beyond what we can bear. As we turn up to work every day, we must remind ourselves daily that we are those jars of clay: fragile and unimpressive. Yet through God's almighty providence, we are pressed (afflicted, in trouble, distressed, or suffering) but not crushed (afflicted to the point of total and complete hopelessness). We are persecuted, but never abandoned by God. We are often struck down, but never destroyed.

So often, work can drive us to the point of being tempted to give up. We consistently walk this fine line between being afflicted and losing all hope. Only by remaining in Jesus the true vine and through the sustenance of the Holy Spirit can we hope to survive this storm. We need to learn to hold fast to Jesus, remembering that though we may be hard pressed from every side, we are not crushed.

For the Junior Doctors

If you are reading this as a junior doctor or medical student, we hope that this book will be more than something you just read through, then leave it on the shelf with the rest of your book collection. This book aims to address some key challenges that will beset a junior doctor when they start work. We hope to provide a solid Christian understanding of work and its various challenges, and to address huge topics which have historically gone unaddressed in the medical field, such as mental health, attitudes, balance, direction, and mentoring.

We hope that beyond learning from the content in this book, you will use this as a tool to initiate a mentorship relationship with a mature Christian adult who can help to support you spiritually and cover you in prayer. Many of us enter the workforce with no mentor or older figure to guide us through the tumultuous journey that we will embark on. We hope that all readers of this book can approach an older Christian doctor and form a one-on-one or small group setting to walk with you through this journey. This book could be used as a guide or a conversation starter, which ideally would prompt deep discussion, edifying mutual encouragement, and confession and prayer. Our hope is that this consistent, godly discourse will lead all readers to become mature Christian doctors who work faithfully with their hands and glorify God with their lives. In time to come, these readers should go on to positively influence other junior doctors and bless them in similar ways.

We will all face many challenges at work, and we will have questions that are specific to us and require individualised and contextual information. Use this book to guide and frame your thoughts and as a tool to explore the difficult topics that tend to plague junior doctors. We want this to be a facilitation tool to raise up these issues to a spiritual mentor who can provide advice, experience, and perspective. In that sense, this material should not limit your discussion and sharing, but merely guide it.

For the Senior Doctors

If you are reading this as someone who has been in the profession for some time, we encourage you to consider being a source of wisdom and love for those who have come after you. Perhaps you have great stories of how God has brought you through as you toiled in your workplace and helped you overcome challenges. You may also have failures and negative examples of your time in medicine. Either way, we are sure that if you are willing to step down to mentor and disciple your juniors, God is capable of using your experiences—both big and small—to speak words that bring encouragement to them.

Even if you have never mentored someone before or feel like you are not suitable as a spiritual leader to anyone, we ask that you prayerfully avail yourself to others who might just need a listening ear. Perhaps as you open your heart to share, you can start to process how you faced the challenges at your work, and eventually wield them as a force for good.

Creating a culture

More than the individual relationships between mentors and mentees, we hope that this book will encourage a strong culture of Christian mentorship within the medical field. The culture of secular mentorship and teaching within this field is already present, and it would be invaluable for us to build a similar culture that builds up the spiritual walks of our Christian junior doctors. A culture of mentorship will need to be built one relationship at a time, with those who have gone before looking back to help those that come after them grow. This certainly will not happen overnight, but instead will be a gradual process that takes place over years to come. Medical work will not immediately become easier, but if we collectively continue to take part in such relational ministry within the workplace, we can continue to build up one another. We hope that our brothers and sisters will not only maintain their faith but grow in faithfulness in their junior doctor years. For the non-believers around us, we pray that they will see the actions and faithfulness of followers of Christ, and God-willing, come to Christ themselves.

There are already a lot of Christian doctors, and so many Christians enter medical school every year. But so many of us become lost or severely discouraged when we start work. If we learn to invest heavily in this culture of mentorship and perpetuate it, we can transform the medical field from what it is now to a place where not only physical healing takes place, but where doctors and other healthcare workers come to know Christ and show His love to the world, just as He has commanded us. Let us start to strive towards this goal, where we can collectively be known as a group of people who serve God, loving Him with all our hearts, souls, minds, and strengths.

PART 1: THEOLOGY OF WORK

WHY DO WE WORK? – GOD'S DESIGN AND REDEMPTION OF WORK

We all know the story: Rachel is rudely woken up by her alarm clock. She washes up in a daze. She feels like she still hasn't recovered from the multiple overnight calls this past week, but she has no choice. She calls for a cab because the trains and buses don't run this early in the day. At the hospital, she sits down at a desk and sighs as she turns the computer on. "I'm so tired. Why am I even doing this?" she says to herself while waiting for her computer to start up. Once it starts, so does her workday, and Rachel loses herself in the unrelenting flurry of activity. The day is filled with treating patients, tasks to do, attending to requests from co-workers or patients. Finally, when work is finished, she picks up her bag and walks out of the hospital, exhausted. The sky is dark, and she is already late for dinner. She books a cab again using her phone, and in the few minutes it takes to get a ride, she thinks to herself, *"What is all of this even for? Where am I going with all this slogging? Why is work so tough? And when am I even going to catch a break?"* A tinge of regret or sadness slowly creeps in, as the sneaking suspicion that she might have chosen the wrong career starts to grow in her heart. But the arrival of her ride cuts off her train of thought. After dinner, she is so exhausted that she cannot really find the will to make plans with friends, catch up with family members, or even to pray. She falls asleep soon after and the routine repeats.

Rachel is a fictional junior doctor. But Rachel's story is the same as so many of ours. She represents the average junior doctor in our medical system: exhausted, questioning her career, possibly jaded, constantly wondering why we work so hard, and what is the end goal of it all. Asking these questions are not a bad thing. In fact, these questions are crucial to answer if we are to live our lives doing God's will.

So, why do we work as a doctor? Perhaps some of us were once enamored with the prospect of changing and saving lives, and so we worked extremely hard to get to where we are. Perhaps some of us were persuaded by family members and friends to enter this respectable and stable profession. Still, some of us might have pursued it because we genuinely thought that God has called us to serve Him in this capacity.

Far from being a human-created construct for the purpose of capitalism, work is deeply theological and inextricably connected to our spiritual life, and we as Christian doctors will do well to understand the theology of why we work.

Work is a part of the original creation

The basis of the theology of work stretches all the way back to the start of the Bible, in Genesis 1 and 2. In Genesis 1, we see God working as He creates the heavens and the Earth, and everything else that fills the Earth. In Genesis 2, we see God putting Adam—the man He had created—to work. Here, in the perfect Garden of Eden as God had originally intended, Adam was told to go ahead and work the land and take care of it. Genesis 2:15 says

"The Lord God took the man and put him in the Garden of Eden to work it and take care of it."

Adam was essentially tasked with maintaining the goodness of the garden and was to take charge of all the living creatures which existed there. This is a beautiful image of work, because we realise that at least in part, mankind was created to work towards a purpose and to be a contributing force for good in God's perfect world. Even when Eve was created, it is stated clearly that Eve was to be a helper to Adam, to aid him in the work that God had commanded him to do. This is the theological basis of our understanding that at its core, work (paid or unpaid) was always meant to be part of our purpose on Earth. To create, to care for, and to strive for something good is fundamental to who we are. Work is also one of the ways we come to understand who we are, since it helps us recognise our unique talents and gifts, which are an essential part of our identity.

Made in God's Image

If we have been Christian for some time, we might have heard that we are "made in God's image". This is absolutely true. The first reference of this is seen in Genesis 1:26, where God says:

"Let us make mankind in our image, in our likeness, so that they may rule over the fish in the sea and the birds in the sky, over the livestock and all the wild animals, and over all the creatures that move along the ground."

One of the foremost applications of this is seen in how we mirror God's pattern of working, creating, and being in charge of the things on this Earth. God himself worked to create the heavens and the earth in the six days of creation described in Genesis 1. Mankind bears that image of God, and we are called to work like how God worked. This is unique compared to all creation because mankind is the only creation that God decided to make in His own image, and mankind was the only one to be set apart and given an actual job description. In this context therefore, our work is a sacred task and one of the ways to live as God intended us to live.

Seeing ourselves as being made in God's image can also come in the form of seeing the goodness in our work (in some sense, similar to how God sees His work's goodness in Genesis 1:31). There will be times, especially in medicine, when you see things are truly beautiful and that points to God's goodness; like the time we get to contribute to the healing of a patient's infection or seeing an elderly man walk again after countless hours of caring for and encouraging him. These are not just "part of the job"; these are moments that testify to the fact that God has put us in our current workplace for a purpose. In times like these, we doctors can take joy in the fact that we bear God's image of a healer when we practise medicine, allowing us to be a vessel of God's healing.

Stewards of the Earth

Furthermore, we can see quite clearly that Adam was called not just to work, but to take care and steward all of God's creation. He was not the original creator of all these things, but he was given dominion over all the plants and animals of the garden. We inherit this responsibility as well and are called to steward the areas of influence in our lives.

This concept of stewardship is actually fairly easy to appreciate in healthcare. Given the nature of our jobs, we are called to steward the health and safety of the patients placed under us. Furthermore, we are called to steward the country's healthcare resources. The way we wield our knowledge in conjunction with said resources directly impact people for better or for worse. Even as a "lowly" junior doctor, whether we put in 100% effort or whether we do the bare minimum can make a real difference in the patients' lives. Being meticulous in summarising and thinking through patients' multiple health issues can ensure that optimal treatment decisions are made, longer-term issues are dealt with on top of the pressing immediate issue, and facilitate transitions of care. Spending more time to explain and encourage patients can improve disease understanding, compliance, and ultimately make a huge difference in health outcomes.

The work of our hands contributes evidently to the preservation of life and the protection of those who are otherwise unable to protect themselves. This is a privilege that is very significant and cannot be taken for granted. As doctors (even junior doctors), we steward a certain authority that if used well, gives us extraordinary ability to care and love. However, it is also double-edged in the sense that it is easily abused or neglected.

When we think about work, we need to remember that every time we step into the hospital or clinic to work, we are here to do something that is God ordained and blessed. We are here to wield our influence for the glory of God and to steward the health of people under our care.

When Work became Toil

The realisation that work is good, a part of the perfect creation, and a godly thing to commit our lives to seems to be sharply contradicted by the very real experiences that we face at work. Even though work is sometimes enjoyable and fulfilling, it is often difficult, draining, overwhelming, and even seemingly fruitless. Like the fictional junior doctor Rachel, we find ourselves constantly questioning why is work so hard, and given enough time, disappointment, and bad experiences, we start to consider giving up and running away from it all. Thankfully, the Bible also offers us a theological explanation for why work seems so toilsome, so far away from the vision of a perfect "Garden of Eden" described in Genesis 2.

Perhaps we have heard the story hundreds of times: The devil (in the form of a serpent) tempts Eve to eat the forbidden fruit. Eve offers some to Adam, and he too eats it. This causes the fall of man, and all the consequences that follow. When Adam and Even sinned, the Bible records that God says:

"Cursed is the ground because of you; through painful toil you will eat food from it all the days of your life. It will produce thorns and thistles for you, and you will eat the plants of the field. By the sweat of your brow you will eat your food"

Genesis 3:17b-19a

This means that what was previously God's perfect creation was now to become a painful toil. Mankind was no longer the perfect creation it once was, now tainted by sin and defiance towards God. Work similarly was tainted by sin, and God's punishment towards mankind was that what was once effortless and fruitful will now require "painful toil" for life. The work also would produce "thorns and thistles" alongside the plants of the field that man cultivated for food. Furthermore, it will be through effort and "sweat of [his] brow" that Adam would get his sustenance.

This speaks of a larger picture of how work is for us today. The painful toil written in Genesis 3 is seen in how difficult our work is and how much effort we have to put in. The thorns and thistles represent the frustrations, fruitlessness, and unwanted troubles we face while trying to do our job. We feel this dissonance sharply and it can easily lead to despair if we do not understand the basis of why we feel this way.

The Tension we hold

Therefore, we as Christian workers (whether doctors or not) need to hold these two things in tension. At its core, work is good. Work was created by God and is a natural part of any human's life. We were created to do good work, not to laze around for the entire duration of our lives, and with the work of our hands give glory to God every single day as we strive. However, work does not feel like nor appear to be the paradise it originally was meant to be because it was tainted by man's sin.

This is why we experience hardship at work, why work sometimes seems fruitless and effortful no matter which profession we find ourselves in. We can and often do see goodness and purpose at work, and might even sometimes get a glimpse of God's glory while working. But its beauty is ultimately tainted by sin. Work is often also hard directly because of the sinfulness of man, be it ourselves or the sin of other people whom we interact with. Pride, selfishness, and distrust play a definitive role in making the workplace toxic and discouraging. Throughout the Bible, we see evidence of humans doing unkind things to each other because of the sin in their hearts.

The Redemption of work

However, such a message would be woefully incomplete and will also drive us to despair if we do not recognise the second part to this equation: God had always planned to rescue the world.

Even though the ground was cursed in Genesis 3 because of the fall of man, God started to make a plan of redemption to provide salvation to His people. We see God promise Adam and Eve that in the end, a child of Eve will come to crush the serpent's head, to put an end to the sinfulness of God's people and ultimately return them to Himself. This child of Eve is of course later revealed to be Jesus, the only perfect man to walk this earth, the Messiah who came to save us and redeem us. But Jesus did not *only* redeem our souls and give us salvation through His death and resurrection. He *also* commissioned us and gave us new commands to love and to work towards the spreading of God's good news in all the earth. In freeing us from sin and death, He gave us a new meaning for worship, a new mission in our lives, and a redemption of our work.

The redemption of work is very much like the redemption of man. Before, we worked for man's approval, for money, and for a sense of significance. When Christ came, He taught us (through His disciples) a new way to live. When Christ commissioned His disciples, He gave us a new reason to use our hands: to make disciples of all nations (Matthew 28:19) and to serve Him through service to the hungry and needy (Matthew 25:40). While we wait for Christ to come again, we have this hope that we hold fast to, even though we look around at this fallen world and recognise that it is fallen.

A new mission for work

Glorifying God

First and foremost, when we become Christians, our new mission now is to glorify God at work. In fact, as Christians we need to realise that our very existence is meant to glorify God. This is a fundamental truth of creation in the Bible. In Isaiah 43:7, God refers to His people as "everyone who is called by [His] name, whom [He] created for [His] glory, whom [He] formed and made". In Matthew 5:16, Jesus tells us to "let [our] light shine before others, so that they may see [our] good works and give glory to [our] Father who is in heaven". In 1 Corinthians 10:31, Paul says to us "so, whether you eat or drink, or whatever you do, do all to the glory of God".

This means that every little thing we do in every aspect of our lives, we hold in high regard as an act of worship to our King. Since we are called to be living sacrifices (Romans 12:1), our entire lives (including eating, drinking, resting, and working) is worship. Worship and glorifying God is our response to God's character and the recognition of the work He has done for us.

If we are called in the middle of the night to insert an intravenous cannula, we insert it to the glory of God. If we have to do a manual disimpaction on a geriatric lady, we do the best disimpaction we can to the glory of God. If we have to talk to that infuriating family member, then we speak in love and use our words to the glory of God. We are so used to thinking that worship equates to singing nice songs with a talented band in an air-conditioned auditorium, we forget that in all the moments we wish we are doing something else, we are still worshipping God through our actions.

Making Disciples of All Nations

When Jesus ascended to heaven, He made sure to tell His disciples what their purpose was. They were to make disciples of all nations, baptising them in the name of the Father, and of the Son, and of the Holy Spirit (Matthew 28:18–20). We as Christians are here on this Earth in order to spread the good news of Jesus to all nations, wherever God calls us to go, and wherever we find ourselves. Our very purpose as we live and breathe is to bring others to know Jesus.

This mission does not stop when we turn up at work. In fact, most of us reading this would spend the majority of our time at work. We have never been told by the Bible that evangelism stops when we are in our paid jobs. Neither are we meant to preach God's Word only in cell groups or on Sundays. We are meant to live with an overflow of love to all around us. And since doctors spend so much time in the hospital/clinics, this is therefore our mission field by default.

To be clear, overtly forcing religious views onto patients should not be done. Doing so might not be well received or worse—might push people away from the gospel. But there are still many things that can be done. It is possible to pray for patients whom we know share our faith. We can even privately pray for those who do not share our faith. We go to hospitals daily, and so tend to forget that this might be the most difficult time of a patient's life. Whether we pray with them or we pray privately for them, we still edify and bless them.

Furthermore, many of our fellow colleagues are Christian. Like us, they might be struggling very hard with fatigue, mental health issues, and stress. We can reach out to them, help them tangibly, and pray for them. Making disciples also involves building up and supporting our fellow brothers and sisters in Christ. If all the Christians in the workplace learn to love and serve each other, we can powerfully support each other in these struggles.

Our actions, words, and deeds also serve as a clear testimony to those who are not currently believers. Our non-Christian colleagues will witness how we work, our attitudes when we show up, and the words and tone we use with others. We are Christ's ambassadors. We do not stop being ambassadors once overnight call starts, nor do we get to choose when to turn on our "Christian mode" in front of others. God can use you to speak into the lives of others, either directly by the sharing of the good news of Jesus, or indirectly as a picture of what a follower of Christ looks like. As we choose to pick up our cross every day, we choose to follow Him. We carry the good news of the saving work of Christ with us in our fragile and imperfect human bodies, like the precious treasure in the ordinary jars of clay described in 2 Corinthians 4:7–10. We can choose to love as He commanded us to, evangelise as He sent us to do, and glorify God in all the work of our hands.

Freedom at work

We need to have eternity in mind and see our entire lives in the lens of Jesus' finished work on the cross. If we forget that Jesus saved and called us for eternity, we will fall into the trap of being very myopic with our purposes. We become pitifully short-sighted and can only think of the next holiday, next paycheck, or next promotion. We end up either working to survive or to prove our worth to other people. This is a trap which often becomes a prison of our own making. We sinful humans easily forget the glorious alternative: that we work to save lives and to save souls as commanded by Jesus, Lord of our lives. Only with this eternal perspective can we gain the proper understanding of work, which leads to newfound freedom in the workplace.

While we are saved through Christ, we recognise that work feels like absolute toil because we still physically live in a fallen world. We work the same ground that was cursed because of Adam and Eve's sin. But we simultaneously need to work while holding fast to the hope of Christ, knowing that we remain here because we seek to glorify God with the work of our hands. We are also placed where we are because we are called to evangelise both with our words and with our lives. We now live in the freedom of Christ. Remembering Christ in our daily work will free us from idolizing anything in the workplace and at the same time free us from becoming idle while at work. It will prevent you from thinking that work can give you everything you ever wanted, and it will also prevent you from thinking about escaping from a job that doesn't matter to God. We are no longer slaves to sin, fear, our bank account, or to our employers. We are given the freedom to choose to be servants of Christ in service of His Kingdom, fighting every day instead to edify others and love God.

The movie "Chariots of Fire" is about two Olympic runners called Eric Liddell (a Christian) and his competitor Harold Abrahams. The movie centers around the story of Liddell, who was a devout believer who chose not to run his race on the Sabbath day out of reverence for God. His friend Harold Abrahams on the other hand, was anxious to win to prove himself. Timothy Keller writes in his book *King's Cross*:

At one point, speaking of the sprint event in which he was competing, [Abrahams] said, "I've got ten seconds to justify my existence."

Liddell, on the other hand, simply wanted to please the God who had already accepted him. That's why he said to his sister, "God made me fast, and when I run I feel his pleasure." Harold Abrahams was weary even when he rested, and Eric Liddell was rested even when he was exerting himself.

Let us be like Eric Liddell, who ran (and eventually won multiple races) with the knowledge that he was doing this for his saviour Jesus. When we work, we aim to please Jesus too because He has redeemed us and redeemed our work. This way, we can honestly say to others that God made us doctors, and when we practise medicine, we too can feel His pleasure.

Discussion Questions:

1a. Which aspects of your work do you find meaningful? Be honest. Do you see it as a part of God's perfect plan for you? Or do you see it as something to be endured?

b. When you are working, do you feel like you are doing what God intended for mankind to do? Why or why not?

2. When you are at work, do you feel like you are showing the image of God? Why or why not?

3a. In your area of medical practice, in what way might you be a steward of God's creation?

b. What are the barriers preventing you from being a good steward?

4. Read Genesis 3.

How does Genesis 3 help to frame how you see your challenges at work?

5. Each of us have motivations or purposes that keep us going at work. What are some of these for you?

6. What opportunities do you have to be a blessing at work?

7. Take some time to reflect on the freedom we have gained from believing in Jesus. How can we remind ourselves of this truth daily?

Pressed But Not Crushed

WHAT DO WE REALLY WORSHIP? – IDOLATRY AND IDLENESS

Idolatry – When one worships medicine

We all know that guy. Brian was the star Christian student in medical school. He led the Christian Fellowship, played the piano in worship, and went for medical missions all the time. He was also the model student, completing all his assignments on time and scoring top marks in every exam. He even spent his spare time helping his classmates. He was pleasant, well liked, and respected amongst the Christian medical community. But something changed when Brian started work. He was always interested in pursuing orthopaedics as a specialty and had done some research as a medical student. Now, he was fully immersed in it as an orthopaedics resident and spends all his time either working hard to impress his seniors or attending socials with his orthopaedic colleagues. When he is home, he is grinding out his 30th research publication on the latest hip surgery technique. He has no time for friends or family anymore and no longer goes to church. When asked how he is doing, Brian is still cheerful and optimistic but only ever talks about career advancement or salary. Occasionally, Brian wonders if he should pray more or do his quiet time. He then proceeds to say a quick 30-second prayer before bed. After all, God will forgive him because he's doing an important conference presentation the next day.

Many (if not all) of us came into medicine liking and even loving the idea of being a doctor. We might not all be like Brian, but we have a certain propensity to get lost in our work and to forsake everything else. Practising medicine has a certain attractiveness to it that inspires so many young, bright-eyed students to compete for those few spots in medical school every year. However, some of us end up placing medicine as the all-important thing in our lives. It ends up becoming the thing with which we build our entire lives around—the foundation on which we build our identity. It ends up becoming an idol in our lives.

Borrowing from Timothy Keller's deeply insightful book *Counterfeit gods*, we can define idols as "anything more important to you than God, anything that absorbs your heart and imagination more than God, anything you seek to give you what only God can give". Basically, anything which we as Christians place above God in terms of hierarchy in our lives. Anything else besides God that we allow to shape our identities and our lives around, and that we turn to for confidence and safety. This can take the form of many

Medicine as an idol

Medicine is especially easy to idolize because of the nature of the work. First of all, we are no longer called Mr, Miss, or Mrs so and so. We are now addressed as Dr once we pass medical school and become a junior doctor. Next, medicine (especially at a junior level) is so demanding in terms of both time and energy that we spend all our waking moments in the hospital trying to do our job well. We then spend all our other moments in our day recuperating and preparing ourselves to go back and perform as best we can at the hospital. Our energy and attention are similarly fully directed at our medical careers. Since medical school, the majority will need to dedicate much of their willpower to cramming as much medical knowledge as possible into their heads, churning out research to impress those in the specialties of our choice, and grabbing as much clinical experience that we can. Junior doctors spend nearly all their willpower trying to survive, much less thrive at work.

Our social circles also start to evolve. Our friend groups are formed predominantly by people in medicine. We speak about medicine in our spare time and casual conversations. Even our language changes to incorporate medical jargon (whether intentionally or not). Our mentors that we look up to in life tend to be senior doctors who have gone before us and achieved much.

With such demands, it is easy to see how so many of us will insidiously start to let medicine become the utmost power in our lives. Every aspect of our lives becomes saturated with it, and it starts to become this all-encompassing entity that we are subject to. This of course does not happen overnight. After all, it is not as if any of us one day sat down and declared that we no longer worship the God of the Bible and instead will bow down before the god of medicine. Instead, it is like a gentle downward-winding path that is smooth sailing and without resistance.

The Bible often speaks of idolatry using the analogy of marriage infidelity, where God's chosen people are committing adultery against God (Hosea 2:2-5, Isaiah 57:7-17). Yet many of us are so attached to medicine that we jokingly admit to others that 'Yes, I am married to medicine'. We longed to feel loved and affirmed by those in our medical community, and we go to great lengths to ensure that other people in medicine approve of us. In contrast, we feel especially hurt when we are scorned or wronged by them.

The Bible also speaks of idolatry in terms of a master-slave relationship, where we are bound to whoever we worship and must do their bidding. Indeed, many of us do what we are told even for things outside our job scope and even though we might not agree with it. We then sheepishly refer to ourselves as 'slaves to the healthcare system' and refer to our employers (jokingly or not) as our 'masters'.

Many of us started work as doctors with good, altruistic intentions. We started off wanting to do our best for our patients and using the work of our hands to bless others. However, medicine can slowly and insidiously take over our lives. The devil is cunning, hence this sin is almost never blatant and obvious, because most Christians will not be able to tell when it began. Rather, idolatry slowly but surely slips in, corrupts us, and traps us.

Other Common Work Idols

While some of us might not be as enamoured with medicine, there are other common traps when we start work.

Pride

Pride itself can be an idol. There are certain moral high grounds that doctors can take when interacting with people who do not practise medicine. First of all, since our jobs are so essential to society, we can start to take pride in the "indispensability" of our occupation. We start to think of ourselves as more important than others and our time being more precious than others'. We can also start to take a certain pride in the difficulty of our jobs. Because it is so demanding in terms of time and energy, we might start to glory in the suffering we so readily undertake. We might even take to boasting to others how many hours we put into our job, expecting affirmation and praise for undertaking that sacrifice daily. Unfortunately, many of us easily take pride in the work that we do, and start to see ourselves as superior beings, at least in the workplace. We slowly forget that we are co-labourers with Christ and our fellow Christians and start to place ourselves above others. As Timothy Keller mentioned in his book *Every Good Endeavor*, it is much easier to feel superior as a doctor than a stockbroker.

Power

Furthermore, power can be another idol in our workplace. Many of us crave control over situations in our lives, and to a certain extent, over other people as well. Becoming a doctor often means that there are situations where you rightly need to take charge. However, that kind of power can become very addictive, especially as we advance in our medical careers and come to expect that kind of power over other people. Furthermore, the power and ability to save lives can give us a sort of god complex at the same time. We can inadvertently start to worship and repeatedly pine for such influence over others, wanting them to do what we say in the way that we want it. It can be seen in some senior doctors who expect junior staff to do things their way and may try to exert power over others in an unedifying way. As junior doctors, we are in danger of emulating such behaviour, or even desiring such power since we do not yet possess it. If we are not careful, the motivation for our careers will slowly start to change. Almost imperceptibly, our priorities will start to centre around the pursuit of such power and influence, forgetting that we practise medicine as envoys sent by God to serve others instead of being served.

Money

Money can also easily become an idol. Doctors get paid a fair amount, depending of course on the type of work and the specialty training of that individual. In an environment where some career paths are better renumerated than others, it can be tempting to start placing money as our guiding light in our medical careers. Jesus mentions the temptation of money more than any other vice in the gospels. This is because He knew that our human hearts are greedy and are often captivated by wealth. Again, it is insidious because many of our conversations will centre around renumeration and potential pay. Be it about working as a locum versus being hired full time, or working in the public sector versus the private sector, we invariably start to weigh options based on how much money we can get. While renumeration is a fair consideration in career planning and in itself is not sinful, a repeated lust for more instead of looking to God for direction on where we are headed tends to start us on a downward spiral. Soon, we no longer work to honour Christ; we work to appease our heart's desire for wealth.

The Problem with idols

Idols are not harmless however. They, like the pagan gods of old, always demand sacrifices from us. In the ancient biblical times, pagan idols demanded things like gold and silver, animal offerings, and even child sacrifices. We may scoff at ancient worshippers for being foolish. However, modern idols are not that much different. In our pursuit of our idols' approval and blessing, we sacrifice our time, energy, and resources. In pursuit of career advancement and prominence in the workplace, we sacrifice our family, our children, friendships, and even our very own bodies on the altar of success. We pay a heavy price as we bow to these modern Gods much like those in the past who used to bow to figurines of animals carved out of precious metals.

The funny thing about worshipping something is that we will never get enough of it. For those who worship money, they will never reach a point where they are satisfied with their current wealth. There is always a higher goal to attain, a better lifestyle to rise to, a new rung of the socioeconomic ladder they need to reach that promises to give us that elusive sense of joy and satisfaction. We will always feel like we don't have enough money. For those who might worship power, no matter how much influence or say we might have over others, it will not satisfy us because there is always someone higher in rank than us. Even if we achieve the highest rank possible in our organisation, someone else might wield more power or influence than us. No matter what, it is not enough. This applies for things outside medicine too. Even those who worship the idea of physical beauty and pursue it wholeheartedly will always see their imperfections in the mirror and feel like they need more beauty.

Returning to God

All of us are guilty of idolatry at some point of time. If not at work, then in our personal lives or in our church ministries. We need to constantly reflect on the condition of our heart and to honestly ask ourselves if we are idolizing something by placing it above God in terms of importance. We need to respond in repentance and give up these idols, actively renouncing them.

However, if we find that we are letting other things rule the throne of our lives, we cannot just recognise and dethrone said thing and think that that is the end of the issue. A power vacuum will always be filled, and something else will take its place as the most important thing in our lives. For example, many of us might fall into the trap of giving up the idol of lofty career goals to be a top cardiac surgeon, only to replace it with idolising how much money we earn per hour working as a locum doctor and "living the luxurious life".

Instead, the answer to the problem of idolatry is returning to God. We need to actively place Jesus as our Lord and Saviour over our lives, and this means placing Him on that throne that was just vacated by our idol. Instead of letting medicine or any or idol shape our lives, we let Jesus and the pursuit of His commands shape all our decisions. We need to cultivate an insatiable desire for God's Word and seek to shape our lives around our service to him.

By enthroning Jesus in our lives and worshipping Him daily, we will find that (like the other idols) we will never have enough of His goodness, and we have to keep pursuing Him all our lives. The key difference here is that Jesus alone promises that He is the way, the truth, and the life. Yes, following Him likewise demands the sacrifice of our whole lives as we become living sacrifices dedicated to God (see Romans 12). But the difference here is that what we get in return is not the slow destruction of our lives, but the restoration of our souls and the promise of salvation and eternal life, blessing on Earth and in heaven, and to always have the presence of God with us.

As we turn up to work each day, let us be mindful of the things that motivate us to do the things we do. When we wake up at ungodly hours to commute to work, we should constantly question ourselves: Who or what am I doing this for? Why do I put myself through this? Do I want to achieve fame, fortune, and respect from other people? Do I do this so my family can be proud of me? Or do I truly want to serve God with all my heart, soul, mind, and strength?

This is a question that is hard to answer and requires absolute raw honesty with ourselves. In the first place, following God is not a matter of 'trying harder' either. We are called to simultaneously strive to serve God yet recognise that we are wholly reliant on God's Holy Spirit to actually serve Him. Furthermore, it will not be a one-off question. It will be one that needs to resurface constantly, especially as we climb the hierarchy where new idols (or the same idols in different forms) await us. We need to constantly come back to our accountability groups and mentors and work through our human tendencies to place idols on pedestals and to be unfaithful to God. If we have close brothers and sisters in Christ in the medical field, then we must also help to look out for them and ask them these hard questions to watch out for them, to love them, and to sharpen them (Proverbs 27:17).

Idleness - When we couldn't care less

John has worked as a junior doctor for four years. During medical school, he aspired to become the best cardiologist that he could be. He wanted to glorify God by saving lives and had dreams of advocating for the underprivileged families in the country. However, the past four years have not been easy on him. Setback after setback had battered him as he failed to get into residency and has been underperforming at work due to a mix of anxiety and fatigue. Recently, he admitted to becoming jaded and has decided that he could not care anymore. He will do his dues as a medical officer and nothing more. Even better, if he could get away with avoiding certain duties in order to leave the hospital early, he would. He delegates as much work as he possibly can and does not care about his colleagues or patients. He spends his workdays on social media and crafting a plan to leave the hospital system for good.

John's story is not unique. Many of us become jaded due to the difficult conditions we face in our work, and we start to develop a sense of laziness and lethargy. There are specific reasons why one might end up working like John, doing just the bare minimum or 'quiet quitting'. Some of us realise that doing more does not lead to more benefits (such as renumeration or recognition), but instead comes at a personal cost. Others might realise that nobody will realise if we are doing more or less at our work. Still others might simply not find any meaning in the profession, realising that it is 'just a job' to earn our wages.

The book *The Gospel at Work* by Sebastian Traeger and Greg Gilbert helps us explore the apparent polar opposite of the sin of idolatry: the sin of idleness. The Bible specifically identifies idleness as a form of sin against God. For example, Paul writes to the Thessalonians:

> *"When we were with you, we told you that if a man does not work, he should not eat. We hear that some are not working. But they are spending their time trying to see what others are doing. Our words to such people are that they should be quiet and go to work. They should eat their own food. In the name of the Lord Jesus Christ we say this. But you, Christian brothers, do not get tired of doing good."*
>
> 2 Thessalonians 3:10–13

Paul has strong words for those who are idle, that they 'should not eat', and that they 'should be quiet and go to work'. This message to the Christians in Thessalonica emphasizes Paul's strong teaching that Christians should not be marked by their inactivity, and that work is meant to be a part of a Christian's life.

Like idolatry, we have some modern-day equivalents of idleness in our workplace. These can take the form of actions that we do, and things we purposefully choose to omit. Deeper down however, it is most evident in our attitudes towards our work. It can be overt, like deliberately doing as little as possible; or it can be subtle, like concluding that work does not matter and viewing it as a necessary evil for which we gain money to support our "real life" and "real ministry".

Colossians 3:23–24 also states:

"Slaves, obey your earthly masters in everything; and do it, not only when their eye is on you and to curry their favor, but with sincerity of heart and reverence for the Lord. Whatever you do, work at it with all your heart, as working for the Lord, not for human masters, since you know that you will receive an inheritance from the Lord as a reward. It is the Lord Christ you are serving."

Paul is telling the Christians in Colossae (in particular the Christians who are slaves) to do their work with sincerity of heart and reverence for God. They are not to do it only when they know that they are being watched, but even when they know that no one is watching and they may not be rewarded for their good deeds. He ends off verse 24 emphasizing again that while in your workplace, even if you are a literal slave, you need to recognise that it is the Lord Christ you are serving. Paul does not just point out 'lack of work' as idleness, but also specifically targets those who are doing 'something' but not with sincerity of heart. This is a calling and hard to achieve by ourselves. But as with all forms of sanctification, we have the Holy Spirit to point out and convict our hearts of the wrongdoing that we are committing. But more importantly, the Holy Spirit works in our hearts, and He changes it more and more into one that is Christ-like.

Examining our attitudes

An important question therefore that we need to ask ourselves is: how have we become idle at our work? And even if we genuinely think that we have not become idle at our work, we need to search our hearts and be wary of becoming idle in our workplace. The sin of becoming idle is reflected best in our attitudes, and our attitudes reflect the condition of our hearts. Certain attitudes which we might hold will reveal a spirit of idleness in how we work.

Actively doing the bare minimum

As junior doctors, we are often inundated with ridiculously large quantities of work to complete. Often, we find ourselves trying to dodge more responsibilities and avoid getting piled up with more work than we already have. We find ourselves purposefully doing just enough so that we are not accused of being negligent, but we are careful not to draw attention to ourselves lest we end up receiving more work because the bosses think we are that efficient and excellent. It is a well-known phenomenon that those who are recognised as being good at their work often find themselves with more work, as superiors would rather give tasks to excellent workers rather than lousy or mediocre ones. As a response, we instinctively start working with 'calculated mediocrity'. Purposefully not putting in effort in order to slip under the radar yet not putting in our best. Doing this might sound like the intelligent thing to do, but unfortunately goes against the command that Paul gives to us in Colossians 3:23–24, where he calls us to work with sincerity of heart and reverence for God. This attitude is not congruent to the beliefs and convictions of the follower of Christ, and hence would be a marker of idleness in our lives should we choose to hold on to such an attitude.

Thinking of work as a 'necessary evil'

Some of us might not purposefully 'slack off' in our workplace but might instead take the attitude that work is a necessary evil. We might treat work like how we treat the queue at the airport departure before we leave on a holiday to Europe: dreary, annoying, and time-consuming but necessary in order to achieve the enjoyment that comes after. We see work as a transaction that enables us to achieve the means we need to live the life we want when we are not working. We as Christians might even see paid work as purely something that provides us with the funds to enable and support Christian ministry.

However, this attitude can be dangerous because it will eventually open the door to us actively resenting our work and treating it as a chore. This again is not congruent with the way that God has designed the human race. As mentioned in the earlier chapter, we were designed to work as image bearers of God. Man was always meant to work the ground and be productive to the glory of God. Even in God's perfect Garden of Eden, Adam was called to do work and shape the world around him. While not everyone is called to paid work (e.g., homemakers, volunteer workers, missionaries), those of us in said work are certainly called to honour God where we are planted. To resent work and treat it as a necessary evil easily brings us to idleness, where we are tempted to stop honouring God with the work of our hands.

Walking away from a call from God

Idleness or laziness can take the form of direct disobedience to God. Sometimes, we as Christians may receive a firm and clear calling from God to do a certain task, very much like the judges or prophets of the Old Testament. However, a number of us might choose to follow in the example of Jonah and run in the opposite direction. Jonah was a prophet who was told by God to go to Nineveh, the capital of the Assyrian empire, to preach repentance to the king. Instead, he ran in the opposite direction to modern day Spain, trying to sail to the other end of the known world so as to escape God's call. He might have been scared of the call, or he might not have liked the idea of allowing the city to repent and receive God's mercy. He might not have thought that it was possible to achieve either. Whatever the reason, he continues to stand as a prime example of disobedience to God's call.

Sometimes we are convicted by God to reach out to a particular person, or to do something to help a patient or a co-worker at the expense of ourselves. This can be an incredibly simple task, or it could be something that requires great effort on our part. For example, we may realise that a particular patient or family member is very distressed. We might at the same time realise that we are in a position to help counsel that person, but we choose not to because doing so will make us end work at a later time or feel more drained than we already are. Another example could be when we are asked to take up a certain administrative role such as a roster planner or take charge of a particular presentation, taking up precious time at home. It could even be that God calls us to a particular career within or outside of medicine, changing the plans we want to have for ourselves.

Many of us are like Jonah in the sense that when the Holy Spirit convicts us to do certain things, we choose not to do so, whether it is due to our own personal reasons, circumstances, perceived limitations, selfishness, laziness, or even fear. This form of disobedience can be witnessed in our daily lives, where we are resistant to the prompting of the Holy Spirit, when we use our human judgement or desires to decide or guide what we do in the workplace.

Idolatry and idleness can co-exist

It is important to realise that idolatry and idleness are not mutually exclusive to each other. Even though they might seem like polar opposites, they can coexist in the same person and shape how he might go about his daily life. It is entirely possible for someone to pine after money and great wealth, seek to climb the corporate ladder and gain power, yet still actively do the bare minimum work and be lazy and selfish.

As Christians we are called to work with sincerity of heart, at the same time realising that we work for the God of the universe, not for ourselves. As people who live in a fallen world, we must realise that we will be tempted to worship other idols, and we will be tempted to laziness and selfishness as well.

We have to be honest with consistently questioning ourselves on why and how we do our work. Do we see work as something to just "power through" and a medium to exchange time for money? Or do we see ourselves as vessels of blessing, working for the one true King? Medical work is not easy and even if we are not being idle at the moment, changes in life circumstances or simply becoming more burnt out can slowly lead us down that path. If we think that we face such a sin, we should constantly speak to one another and help each other to honour God with both our hands (work) and our hearts (attitudes).

The writer of Hebrew calls us Christians to do just this. He writes in Hebrews 10 that since we have confidence from Jesus' death and resurrection, we should encourage each other to do good deeds. Hebrews 10:23–25 goes:

"Let us hold unswervingly to the hope we profess, for he who promised is faithful. And let us consider how we may spur one another on toward love and good deeds, not giving up meeting together, as some are in the habit of doing, but encouraging one another—and all the more as you see the Day approaching."

As we meet in our accountability groups, or as we see each other in the corridor of the hospital each day, do not let the opportunity pass by ignoring each other or simply lapse into a complaining session. Instead, use the time to spur one another on towards love and good deeds!

Discussion Questions: Idolatry

1. Are there any potential (or definite) idols in your life now? (I.e., Anything that you are tempted to love more than God?)

2. Why do you think is it so easy to idolize medicine as a career?

3. Why are idols harmful to us? Why does God call us to give them up?

Confess about personal idols. Pray for each other, that we will give up our idols and place Jesus at the throne of our lives.

Discussion Questions: Idleness

1. Was there ever a time you did less than you should have? What was in your mind at the time?

2. When you feel that work is dreary and you want to just do the minimum, what do you say to yourself?

3. How can you encourage other Christian doctors to work hard for God?

Confess the times you have been lazy or idle. Pray for the Holy Spirit to enable you to do your best work for the glory of God every day.

PART 2: WORK AND OUR LIVES

WORK-LIFE-FAITH BALANCE

The question of work-life balance is a pertinent one in all professions. However, medicine is sometimes uniquely demanding in this respect. The combination of long working days, lengthy calls, professional exams, and residency often culminates in a work schedule that seems incompatible with life in general. For Christian doctors, we tend to face the Work-Life-Faith Balance problem. We simply add one more factor into our equation and try our hardest to balance it out, praying for the strength to do it all. Most often though, this ends up failing, and we live in a constant cycle of being extremely busy but never really feeling like we fulfil the requirements of any of these three things. We might even feel trapped by the differing "demands" and get the sense that we are not "performing" up to standard.

We all respond in different ways to being stretched in so many directions. Some of us stop having a life outside of work and decide to drop many important aspects of our Christian faith in order to focus on our careers. Some of us try to work as hard as possible when we can, in the hopes that one day when we reach some arbitrary stage in our careers or earn enough money, we can take it slow. Nowadays, an increasing number of individuals choose to prioritise families and free time over work and try to do the minimum work we possibly can. These courses of action are not explicitly wrong. But perhaps as a Christian junior doctor, we really need to evaluate these decisions through a completely different lens than our non-Christian counterparts.

Christ changes how we work

Christ changes how we do everything. His life, His teachings, and ultimately His death and resurrection have enormous implications as to how we see our lives. Our work is no exception. In John 6:27, Jesus tells His disciples "not to work for the food that perishes, but for the food that endures to eternal life, which the Son of Man will give" to us. This means that Jesus actually calls us to labour, but not for our daily wage or public recognition. He calls us to put in the work for things that have eternal value, that ultimately can only be given by Him alone.

The Christians of the New Testament were never called to stop working, and many books of the New Testament assumes and commends the dignity of work. In fact, Paul writes in Ephesians 4:28

"Anyone who has been stealing must steal no longer, but must work, doing something useful with their own hands, that they may have something to share with those in need".

He commands us to work not just so that we will have enough to eat, but so that we can help others who are in need. Yes, it is biblical and God-honouring to work for our living (2 Thessalonians 3:10). However, we are called to work for more than ourselves.

John Piper comments about work in his podcast 'Ask Pastor John' on the episode 'How does Christ Change the Way I Work?': *"Christ dominates your mind as the supreme treasure... So, you go to work not dominated by the desire for the bread that perishes or for the fear of losing it. You go to work knowing him, trusting him, treasuring him, being satisfied in him with your heart set on making much of him. That's how you go to work now. He's dominant in your mind. He's dominant in your heart. And every aspect of your vocation becomes a way of magnifying him."*

Christians are not called to be balanced

Christians are called to view life differently from the world too. A non-Christian will understandably try to hold both work and life in a constant tension, like trying to balance something on a fulcrum or dividing up a pie. A Christian caught up in the pursuit of work-life-faith balance might likewise try to do the same with all three. This is not the way we are called to view our lives. The Bible does not call us to view faith, work, and life as three desirable objects to have and maintain ownership over. We are not called to weigh each of these equally and try to hold them in tension. They are simply not of equal value, nor of the same substance.

Furthermore, the Bible never calls us to be balanced at all. God's Word does not ever promise that spiritual maturity will bring a sense of constant balance between our personal lives and our faith. Instead, the Bible calls us to single-minded devotion to our faith in Jesus (Hebrews 12:1–2); we are called to be Christ-like. Jesus was not balanced—in His "career" as a teacher (or "rabbi"), He was wholeheartedly doing the will of God. He consistently travelled where God called Him to in order to preach the gospel. He obeyed God in all of life and work, even obeying Him to the point of death. Likewise, His disciples were not balanced either. Paul, Peter, and John all lived life according to how God called them, pursuing their faith relentlessly at the cost of their careers, societal standing, and ultimately their lives.

Instead, we are called to work and live for God. Work and life are not opposites to be balanced on a scale. Both are integral parts of our existence, and both are tools which we use to glorify God. In Genesis, work is a part of the perfect creation, not something to resent or fight against (see chapter on the theology of work). When there was no sin in the world, God breathed life into man and set him to work on the Earth. Man was not to work or live for wealth, fame, recognition, or power. Instead, he was to honour God, to live in His image, and to steward the earth well.

Christ-Centeredness

Instead of pursuing work-life balance, we should strive to pursue Christ-centeredness. This means that we commit to placing Jesus at the center of our lives, and then design and manage all the different parts of our lives around that center. As high-achieving, intelligent individuals, junior doctors inadvertently are tempted to live as though we ourselves are the very center of our lives. We tend to focus on our jobs, our relationships, our achievements, our money, and our self-worth. We forget that the Bible tells us the solution to the human condition is to live Christ-centered lives. We then wonder why our self-centeredness has gotten our lives all out of whack.

Therefore, the challenge is not to balance or juggle our faith, our lives, and our work. The challenge is to consistently place Christ at the center of all we do. This might mean actively seeing our work and our relationships through the lens of Christ. Doing this might end up looking like sacrificing rest and family time to save a patient's life or help our fellow colleagues. Or it might involve us actively giving up career opportunities that will tempt us away from following Jesus.

This means that in our everyday lives, the question is not really how many hours we should spend at the hospital, at home, or in church. Instead, every waking moment should present us with the questions: What is the most God-honouring thing I can do right now? And how can I make sure I place Jesus at the center of this situation?

The same concept applies for other crucial things, such as our marriages. For those of us who have spouses, we are called to take the same approach. We do not balance our spouse on one side of a see-saw and our faith on the other, trying to divide our time and affection as equally as possible. Instead, our affections should first and foremost be for God Himself. Consequently, our love for God and our desire to honour and obey Him compels us to love, serve, and submit to and sacrifice for our spouse out of reverence for Christ (Ephesians 5:21–33). Our careers and our lives should be governed by the same principle, where in both scenarios, we are driven by our love for God.

Crucial ways to stay focused

Preaching the gospel to yourself

Many Christian writers[1] repeatedly call for Christians to preach the gospel to ourselves. This is not a new idea, as the psalmist in Psalm 42:5 preaches to his own soul to "hope in God". This might seem counterintuitive. We have the tendency to think that the gospel message is only meant for non-Christians or those who have never heard the good news of Christ. We could not be more mistaken.

The gospel message is key in understanding our identity and setting us free from the many shackles we find ourselves in (sometimes even self-inflicted ones). The gospel message tells us that our original identity is one of a helpless sinner. We were slaves to sin (Romans 6:20), and we had no hope of freeing ourselves. Instead, we needed a Saviour to step down from heaven and redeem us. Now, the gospel calls us to live in light of this newfound freedom, working to serve others and tell them of this freedom you gained.

Thus, the gospel messages tell us our identity: a sinner redeemed for good work. We cannot be prideful or egoistic, because we had no power to even save ourselves. We cannot

---

[1] For example, *The Discipline of Grace* by Jerry Bridges, quoting Jack Miller, a professor at Westminster Theological Seminary

be ashamed, because our ledger was wiped clean before God, and we have no condemnation on us (Romans 3:24). The gospel gives us purpose, because it tells us that the same Jesus who purchased us also sends us out to do good work. We therefore are free to work hard out of love for God, in gratitude for His gifts and a genuine desire to please Him like a child wanting to please their father.

Knowing your life purpose

Another important aspect of this is knowing our purpose of existence. A clear vision of our very purpose is most powerful in excluding what is precisely *not* our purpose. For example, if the medical team knows that the primary purpose for the palliative admission of an end-stage cancer patient is to provide comfort in their limited time left, they will know that sending the patient to the ICU for a painful intubation is not fulfilling the purpose of the admission. In the same way, if we know the purpose of our limited time on Earth, we will not waste time chasing meaningless things that are not aligned with that purpose. As disciples of Christ, our chief purpose is to glorify God, and to enjoy him forever[2]. As we do so, we are commanded to make disciples of all nations (Matthew 28:16–20) and to love others as Christ has loved us (John 13:34). Following Jesus' example, we can learn to

---

[2] Westminster shorter catechism.

live life with overarching purpose which guides all our actions.

Obviously, there will be seasons in life in and out of work. In certain seasons, glorifying God might mean working extraordinarily hard. God might call you to pour all your intellect and time into becoming the best orthopaedic surgeon that you can possibly be. He might call you to the mission field to bless the most disadvantaged people in order to shine His light in a dark place full of suffering. In these situations, honouring God might entail working harder than we have ever worked in our lives. Jesus' season of ministry work was essentially three busy years of travelling to preach the gospel, mentoring His disciples, and ultimately carrying a heavy cross to His death.

In certain seasons, glorifying God might mean that we are called away from our work accolades and potential for advancement. God might call us to become parents or to take care of a sick family member. He might call us out of the medical profession, to pursue other paths that honour Him. Paul held high societal standing, power, and a comfortable life as a pharisee, but he was called away from all these things to be a disciple who lived humbly, was shipwrecked, and imprisoned.

Either way, we are called to discern wisely (and in godly community) which of our choices are more honouring to God. It is possible to pursue career for selfish reasons and call it worship. It is also possible to shun your career for selfish reasons and claim that we are focusing on God.

Discussion questions:

1. How do you currently approach the tension between work, life, and faith? Share your thoughts and personal takes on this issue.

2. Reflect on Ephesians 4:28 where Paul encourages believers to work not only for personal gain but to be able to share with those in need. How can this command challenge us to change how we view work?

3. Reflect on the idea that Christians are called to be Christ-centered instead of "balanced". Do you agree? How does this differ from the conventional understanding of work-life balance?

4. Living a Christ-centered life is easy to say in a book but hard to live out. How can we keep each other accountable in doing this consistently?

5. Discuss practical ways that you can actively place Jesus at the center of your daily life, work, and relationships. Share specific challenges you would face in doing this.

6. What do you think is your life's purpose as a Christian? Try and articulate this and share with each other.

THE JUNIOR DOCTOR AND THE CHURCH

The Christian life is a life lived in community. To be baptized into Christ is to become part of Christ's body on earth, His Church. There are at least 24 "one another" commands in the New Testament (e.g., love one another, honour one another, live in harmony with one another, build up one another). This means that the normal Christian life must be one where we follow Christ in the company of other believers. There are many commands for followers of Jesus to love one another, especially in the gospel of John (John 15:12–17). Most of us belong to a local church as a direct (although not exclusive) embodiment of Christian community.

However, junior doctors face conflicting problems. First of all, junior doctors work long days, mandatory weekend rounds, and exhausting overnight calls. This schedule often clashes with church programmes and activities. At the same time, this transition from student to doctor is especially challenging,. This creates a seemingly impossible problem where the junior doctor is absent from church yet need increasing amounts of spiritual support and nourishment. How do we resolve this conundrum?

Junior doctors: What can you do to not neglect Christian community

We begin by recognizing that our work in the healthcare system is a ministry as well, where we serve God and love those who has been placed in our care. We are called to be citizens of heaven, but we are also called to live in the world and conduct our ministry here. We serve God through evangelism, community outreach, and through service in church. But we also serve God in our work in the hospitals. Since we are called to be Christ ambassadors everywhere we go, and we find ourselves spending most of our time in the hospitals, then the hospitals are our mission field by default. We are called therefore to obey commands to serve, love, and evangelise in this mission field. We need to give time and attention to grow in our expertise in this ministry. This includes taking our training seriously and putting in the necessary time and effort to learn and become excellent at our work- which is doing God's good work where we find ourselves.

Yet, we need to remember that we still have an overall choice to choose how we spend the little time away from work that we have. We will spend time on what we prioritise. In this stage of life we are especially in need of supportive, Christian friendships, and that they play a key role in helping us navigate the most difficult times of our lives while remaining rooted in Christ.

This requires deliberate re-evaluation of how we spend our time. Perhaps there are unedifying and unhelpful things we spend time on in our lives. Perhaps a hobby or our social media page needs to take a backseat for some time in order to preserve our walk with God and our relationships with closest friends and family, while still doing excellent medical work. As such, we might need to step back and re-evaluate how we spend our time and where we place emphases. Arguably, it is not only doctors who face this transitional change. Other demanding professions, new parents, or individuals in busy seasons of their lives will also have to deal with ever-decreasing amounts of time, yet an ever-increasing number of commitments. Where a medical student might be capable of attending multiple gatherings of church and para-church organisations, junior doctors can focus on meeting up with only two or three people once a month for spiritual conversations and to pray together. The focus has to change from one of 'attending Christian events' to one that emphasizes spiritual accountability—the genuine sharing of struggles, vulnerable confession of sin, and radical commitment to serving God in our lives. We are called to walk together after all, encouraging one another on towards good deeds (Hebrews 10:24). Individual circumstances differ and there is no one-sized-fits-all approach. This calls for wisdom on how stay rooted in community and to walk with those who will keep us on the path of life, fighting the good fight together.

Churches: How can we better support our junior doctors?

It is our observation that church communities in Singapore have many times struggled to support our junior doctors. Some frown upon junior doctors missing church services or programmes once they start work, and might question the commitment and spirituality of the junior doctors in their church. But just because a junior doctor cannot attend church regularly for a certain season life does not mean that he or she ceases to belong to the church community or is not committed to glorifying God. Perhaps greater public understanding of the struggles of healthcare workers, as highlighted during the COVID-19 pandemic, might go some way to bridge the divide.

We do not expect to send a Christian missionary to another country without the financial and spiritual support of a home church. Nor do we send out an infantry platoon to battle without artillery support and a route for reinforcements and resupply. Sure, they have to be the ones who are on the frontlines, but they do so with support from behind. In the same way, while our junior doctors who enter the workplace and face the challenges head on, they should not fight this battle alone.

How best can we support the junior doctors? Our churches often swing heavily towards a programme/event-based method of delivering spiritual food to the congregation (a seminar or a lecture, or cell groups that meet weekly). This is certainly not wrong, but in this case, is unsuitable. These ministries are hard to attend regularly when work is fairly unpredictable and sometimes has no fixed schedule week to week. The support that will truly build up our junior doctors will need to come from a more organic and relational ministry, like in the New Testament church.

When Jesus walked this earth 2000 years ago, the primary form of ministry was one of mentorship and discipleship. There was no fixed programme or structure for Jesus to minister to His disciples. He was securely grounded in His relationship with God the Father, and He simply walked with the disciples for years, teaching them whenever the opportunity arose and always encouraging them and rebuking them where appropriate. The New Testament makes no mention of explicit "church programmes", but repeated mentions of simply meeting together to pray, dedicating themselves to the teachings of the apostles, and bearing one another's burdens. Perhaps in this context, we can start to think about emulating Jesus' method of ministry, and the early church's way of doing life. We can start to build junior doctors up spiritually with individual relational ministry that matches their schedules and caters to their needs, and in so doing ensure that this Christian walk is not a solo act, but a team effort done with the combined and perpetual support within the body of Christ.

Spiritual Mentorship in Medicine

We wish to take this chance to advocate for a culture of spiritual mentorship in medicine. We put forth that both within and outside church communities, senior Christian doctors are uniquely placed and have a special duty to support our juniors. Medicine is no stranger to secular mentor-mentee relationships. In fact, medicine is often said to be an apprenticeship, in which juniors learn by emulating their seniors. This is not too different from discipleship in biblical times, which would involve a student or an apprentice living with and having daily interactions with a master, learning their craft by imitation and experience.

Hence, those who have gone before can and should mentor and support those who are currently struggling. Seniors have a special opportunity to inspire junior doctors to become kind, loving, hardworking, and genuine walking testimonies of God's goodness. Even previous negative experiences and suffering can be a blessing in teaching juniors how to better navigate the difficulties in the practice of medicine.

A mentoring relationship is a two-way street and either party can initiate. Juniors can be active in asking for and finding mentors . Senior doctors can offer to mentor believing juniors around them, whether in church or at the workplace. Those who know brothers and sisters who are struggling should gather round such individuals, and perhaps connect them with mentors who can help them through this difficult time. We are not all called to be pastors, but we are all called to pastoral (shepherding) work. We are not all evangelists, but we are all called to make disciples of all nations. We are not all called to be biological parents, but we are all called to be spiritual family members in the family of Christ. Hence, you don't need to have had theological training or experience before you care for someone and share your own experience in order to help them through their tough times. Organic, relational ministry does not have an easy or simple algorithm to follow. It is raw, unguided, and highly subjective. But that is also how we are called to love one another.

Discussion questions

1. Reflect on the commands of the New Testament that relates to loving one another and building up one another. How do these commands shape your understanding of Christian community and its importance in your life?

2. In what ways do the demands of medicine challenge your ability to maintain relationships and belonging in a church community? How can you combat this?

3. How have mentorship and spiritual friendships impacted your journey in the past? How can we provide this for others who come after us?

4. How can you reach out and support friends and colleagues who are going through a rough time in their lives?

DIRECTION AND CALLING IN MEDICINE

Work as calling

Why did you choose to study medicine? Did you feel called to it? Were you pressurised into it by family and friends? Maybe you weren't sure why you chose to pursue medicine. But you survived medical school. Maybe you did well academically. But why medicine? As you embark on your medical career, it's good to revisit this question.

The Callings of God

The primary call of a Christian is not to a particular profession. Our first call is the call to follow Jesus (Mark 8:34–35). We are saved by faith, but we are saved to follow Jesus as our Saviour and Lord. This first calling must be settled first. Once we have decided to follow Christ, we are saying that our lives belong to Him. We are not our own. We were bought with a price.

But there is also a second calling: the call to a particular vocation. God is not into mass production. He made us all unique, with different personalities and strengths and burdens. We follow Christ with our unique selves. God created us with different personal life missions in mind (Jeremiah 1:4–5; Ephesians 2:10). So if we are serious about following God, we need to understand how He has made each one of us and what He has called us to do. To take calling seriously is to understand the need to be good stewards of our lives and our uniqueness.

Clarity as to our calling also has a number of other benefits. It could guide us as we consider postgraduate training. It can help us to persevere when the going gets tough and prevent us from pursuing our career for the wrong reasons, like the pursuit of money and status.

Discovering our calling

If indeed God has a specific mission for us, how do we go about discovering it? Are we called to medicine? If yes, what aspect of medicine are we called to pursue? There are many options in healthcare. Sometimes, like Paul, our callings come in dramatic and unmistakable ways (Acts 9: 1–19). For most of us however, understanding our calling is a lifelong journey of understanding who we are. There are three clues as to our calling.

First, we should consider our primary *ability*. Most of us can do a number of things well but there usually is one or two abilities that stick out. For example, do we work best with our hands (e.g., surgery), or with people (e.g., psychiatry and primary care), or with ideas (e.g., public health policy and research)? We may not be clear earlier in our medical career, but this should get clearer as we go through various career stages and as we are more exposed to the various types of medical work. Some may find themselves better at management than at actual interfacing with patients. Our calling should allow us to be good stewards of what we do best (1 Peter 4:10).

Second, we should consider our primary *burden*. Moses was burdened to see Israel free from slavery in Egypt. Paul was burdened to preach the gospel. There are many needs in our broken world, and medicine addresses many of those needs. To have greater clarity of our calling we should take time to discern which need in a broken world weighs heaviest on our hearts. What need disturbs us the most? What brokenness or lack makes us most angry? What need occupies our thinking the most? Some are burdened to help families at the front lines of medicine. They may end up as primary care physicians or in emergency medicine. Some are burdened to pursue research so there can be new pharmaceuticals, surgical techniques, or biotechnology that can better address some pressing needs. Some have a heart for the elderly and thus are led to geriatric medicine. Some are burdened to comfort the dying and therefore provide palliative care. The list goes on because medicine is broad enough to encompass many areas of concern. As we search for our path within medicine, remember that our calling should allow us to be good stewards of our burdens.

Finally, our calling should make sense of our life *journeys*. As we journey through life, we experience *critical events* that become key transitions that shape our life trajectory. These experiences—what happened, when they happened—are unique to each of us. By examining our personal timelines and experiences, we can be aware of these hinge moments that shape who we are and what we do. If we believe that life is not random and meaningless, but that God authors our lives, we will then look at our lives for clues that will guide us on what we should do and our next chapters. In Genesis 50:20, Joseph told his brothers that they meant to do evil against him by selling him off to slavery, but God meant it for good, to save many lives through his eventual leadership position in Egypt. Like Joseph, we should consider critical events in our lives through the lens of God's sovereignty, and consider that God may be working to guide us to our calling.

The clue to our calling then is our A, B, and C: abilities, burdens, and critical life incidents. How do we discover our A, B, and C? With two basic spiritual disciplines: solitude and community. Doctors are some of the busiest people around, and junior doctors have even less control over their time. Yet, if we are serious about discovering God's calling for our lives, we must carve out times of solitude so we can hear what the Lord may be saying to us. We also need the help of others to help clarify our calling. The heart is deceitful, and we may end up thinking we are hearing from God when it is actually our own desires. Mentors, spiritual directors, disciplers, and spiritual friends can pray along with us and ask the right questions to help us clarify our thinking as to what our calling may be. Discerning companions may also provide needed encouragement and support if one is daunted by what they believe God is calling them to do.

Faithfulness along the way

We take vocation seriously because we want to be good stewards of our lives and our uniqueness. However, for most of us, discovering our calling may take time. Even if we have some clarity about our calling, there may be life circumstances that may prevent us from pursuing our calling at a given point in time. For example, there may be demanding family needs like the care of aged parents or a family member going through a major health challenge that demands our attention. Therefore, while we take our calling seriously, our life is not built around our calling, but around the God who gave us our calling. Hence, while we should endeavour to discover and follow our calling, at any given point in time, we seek the Lord as to what He wants us to focus on. Our ultimate and lasting primary call is to follow Christ and to be faithful to what He wants us to do.

The times when we have to lay aside our calling for a season may still be used by God to shape us for our calling. These could be times when He shapes our character in preparation for when we are to live out our calling. We may be concerned for what we can do for Him. He may be more concerned for what He can do in us first.

Followers of Christ know we are saved by grace not by works. We are saved because we accept God's free gift of salvation. But as people who have been transformed by the gospel, we want to pass forward the grace we have received. One way we can do that is to better understand our vocation and follow it.

Discussion questions

1. Are you a follower of Christ? If yes, what does that mean to you?

2. Do you believe God has a specific calling for you? If yes, what do you think that is?

3. Three clues that may help us understand our calling is understanding our main ability, our main burden, and the key critical incidents of our lives. What would you put down as your A, B, and Cs?

4. What steps can you take to find the solitude and community you need to discover your calling?

5. If you know your calling, is there anything preventing you from pursuing it? Why do you think this is so? What do you think God is up to in this regard?

PART 3: CHALLENGES AT WORK

WHEN WE LOOK AT OUR PATIENTS – ATTITUDES OF CHRISTIAN DOCTORS

As doctors, one of the most important aspects of our work is obviously the patients that comes under our care, whether directly or indirectly. How we think of them directly affects how we treat them and the level of care that we provide to them. When most of us started medical school, we would have spent a lot of time talking about buzz words like "patient-centred care" or "putting the patient first". However, as we start work and become progressively more burdened with the load that comes with the job, we sometimes unwittingly turn this godly calling into a fight for survival and forget our original desire to serve. In our exhaustion we forget that the patients we deal with every day are human beings with intrinsic, irrevocable value. We forget that though this is our daily "bread and butter work", for the patients, being hospitalised is probably the worst time of their life.

Whether or not we take the effort to communicate properly, act kindly, or be patient with them can be the difference between them feeling lost and scared, or feeling reassured and safe. Ultimately, the question we should have is: am I loving these patients as Christ has commanded me, or am I just trying to survive in my job with a "do the minimum then get lost" mentality?

Biblical View of Patients

Many doctors who have grown used to the daily grind of medicine might start to view patients and their issues as obstacles to overcome. They are simply hurdles between us and going home on time. However, this view is unhealthy and not reflective of our view as Christians who are called to love and care for the *"least of these"* (Matthew 25:45), the patients placed under our charge, the ones whose lives have been placed under our stewardship. Our patients are not problems to be solved, nor projects to be worked on. They are God's creation (no matter Christian or not) that are placed in our lives for a time. We are given an exclusive opportunity to bless them with the work of our hands and the words of our mouths.

Many struggle with this because patients and their family can be demanding, rude, entitled, or downright obnoxious. For the most part, we do not find it hard to be nice to people who are nice to us. But we find it exceedingly difficult to put in effort to love those who might go so far as to spit on us and submit formal complaints about us. However, we as servants of Christ must remember that their worst and most apparently ugly traits are not their whole identity. They are God's creation, who have needs and wants. They have had past experiences which has shaped them into the people that they are today. Whether their behaviour is their fault or not, we need to recognise that our call to love, bless, and help does not change when the person we are facing is an absolute thorn in the flesh. Jesus goes so far as to tell us to love our enemies and those who persecute us (Matthew 5:44). He then went and showed us that example on the cross, when He died saving those that insisted on killing Him.

God's Children Made in His Image

Theologically speaking, all our patients (and all of mankind) are made in God's image. The reason why we sometimes cannot visualize that is because sin has come into our lives and tainted this image for all of us. This is why we are waiting to be restored and renewed, and this is why we wait for the last days where we are given new bodies free from the tarnish of sin. Meanwhile, we are to see past (but not overlook) this sin in others and do good to others, knowing that they are precious to God whether we like them or not.

If we are Christians, and if we are to be obedient to God's Word, then we should not even be cursing or speaking ill of our difficult patients with our mouths. James 3:9 clearly explains how doing so is a sin to God. He writes: *"With the tongue we praise our Lord and Father, and with it we curse human beings, who have been made in God's likeness."*

This was a criticism to people who were hypocritical with their worship, whereby they used their tongue to both praise God and speak ill of other people. This criticism is very relevant to us today. If we go to church and sing songs to God on Sunday, but say ugly things about the people who are placed under our charge and their families, we fail to worship God in the way that He desires us to do so. Jesus also expounds on the flipside of this topic in the gospels. Matthew 25:31–46 records Jesus as saying:

"'For I was hungry and you gave me something to eat, I was thirsty and you gave me something to drink, I was a stranger and you invited me in, I needed clothes and you clothed me, I was sick and you looked after me, I was in prison and you came to visit me.'

"Then the righteous will answer him, 'Lord, when did we see you hungry and feed you, or thirsty and give you something to drink? When did we see you a stranger and invite you in, or needing clothes and clothe you? When did we see you sick or in prison and go to visit you?' The King will reply, 'Truly I tell you, whatever you did for one of the least of these brothers and sisters of mine, you did for me.'

"Then he will say to those on his left, 'Depart from me, you who are cursed, into the eternal fire prepared for the devil and his angels. For I was hungry and you gave me nothing to eat, I was thirsty and you gave me nothing to drink, I was a stranger and you did not invite me in, I needed clothes and you did not clothe me, I was sick and in prison and you did not look after me.' "They also will answer, 'Lord, when did we see you hungry or thirsty or a stranger or needing clothes or sick or in prison, and did not help you?'

"He will reply, 'Truly I tell you, whatever you did not do for one of the least of these, you did not do for me.'"

Jesus is saying here that by loving the less fortunate, by serving the sick and the lame, by ministering to their needs, we are ministering to Christ Himself! So, the next time we face a patient or a family member we find difficult to care for, it will be helpful to picture ourselves caring for Christ the King. With this image in mind, we are to do our work well, viewing it as working for our Lord Jesus and not for the man or woman in front of us. This is formative and important also in framing why we do our jobs. It is not merely to please others, but sincerely our acts as living sacrifices for God.

A Privilege to Serve

God is the true healer; the Bible tells us that. We doctors have skills and abilities which we have trained to put into practice so as to serve our patients. However, as Christians we believe that God chooses to use us as His instruments of healing and blessing. In this sense, we are blessed to be invited to be a part of God's will in enacting a plan of healing and restoration of the bodies of other people. This is an immense privilege, and we as doctors get to be in such a unique and valuable position to be a vessel of blessing. This is not something to take lightly. Our title as doctors is not a status symbol. It is an awesome privilege, a power to be wielded with reverence and with humility. As written in Acts 20:35, "it is more blessed to give than to receive".

The Word of God tells us: *"to whom much has been given, much will be required"* (Luke 12:48). Spiderman's Uncle Ben tells us: "with great power comes great responsibility". What we must know is that we are not in this profession just to survive, earn a decent wage, or gain street credibility and respect. Patients are not cash cows which we milk for income. They are precious lives we get to be a part of stewarding. We must be set apart as Christian doctors because we are placed here to serve and to love, and we must remember to bear this responsibility well. We have been given much in many ways. We have been given an abundance of opportunity, support, and position. We then must wield these privileges well and not just for ourselves. Furthermore, though we cannot overtly evangelize to our patients, we can through our service and our kindness show a glimpse of

God's goodness in a time where they are sincerely struggling, sometimes even for their lives.

Discussion Questions:

1. Share a time when you found it challenging to love or serve someone who was very difficult. How did your faith guide your response?

2. How does your understanding of people made in God's image impact the way you perceive and treat others, especially those who are difficult to love?

3. Reflect on your work experience. In what ways do you see your profession as a privilege and opportunity to serve others?

WHEN WE MAKE MISTAKES – OUR RESPONSE TO MEDICAL ERRORS

Linda is a first-year resident in general surgery. While on a night call, she was called in to see a patient who had severe abdominal pain post-surgery. She reviewed the patient and found that though he was in pain, his vital signs were normal, and she did not see any clinical signs that indicated his life was in danger. She proceeds to give him analgesics and moves on with her call. The next day, she woke up post-call to realise that her patient has had an anastomotic leak and is severely ill in the intensive care unit (ICU). A few days later, the patient passed away. Upon finding this out, she doubted herself severely. Her negative thoughts continuously bombarded her. Did she miss something that she should not have? Should she have checked more thoroughly, and perhaps ordered the patient a scan? Is she going to be disciplined for this and lose her job? Is she worthy of being a doctor? Should she even continue practicing medicine? Why is she so useless?

Such situations are not unique, especially amongst junior doctors. There is a distinct fear that we might in our inexperience and fatigue cause harm or fail to prevent the deaths of our patients. We spend our time furiously checking our work, and we feel anxious long after our workday is finished. When things happen and patients are harmed or die, we might blame ourselves or severely doubt our abilities and call to medicine. We are not alone in this struggle. Most, if not all doctors will face this fear, even after they become more senior at work.

We will all make mistakes

Atul Gawande wrote in his book *Complications: A Surgeon's Notes on an Imperfect Science* that "all doctors make terrible mistakes". Ask any doctor who has practiced medicine for some time. He or she can tell you that they have in some form or another made mistakes. Some may have even caused grave patient harm. Some cease to be doctors because of this reason. Many are plagued by the anxiety that we will one day harm our patients. This crippling fear is therefore not something that we should tackle alone, but one that we should address together as a community of Christ-followers. In the same way we are called to work as one that comes from God, we as Christian doctors need to understand life, death, and even unintentional harm in the context of our faith.

Whatever the case, there seems to be little mention in Christian literature about the theological understanding towards medical error. Instead, much of our learnt attitudes toward medical error is coloured by secular ethics, law, patient safety frameworks, and modern culture. This is not necessarily a bad thing. We as doctors function under the rule of law as we practice medicine, and to follow that rule of law is entirely biblical. For example, ethico-legal principles such as open disclosure, as codified in the Singapore Medical Council's ethical code[3], along with local hospital policies and directives constitute one form of governing authority we work under and should be followed dutifully (as set out in Romans 13:1-5). Beyond this secular response, which this book is not able to cover in full, we also need to face the situation of medical error in the same way as any other difficult scenario: through the lens of our faith – as imperfect, fallible sinners saved only by grace.

Not All Medical Errors are the Same

It can be tempting to think in a rather dichotomous manner when we face tough situations, such as patient harm resulting from the actions of the treating team. We tend to either think that there was an error made, or there was none. However, medical errors are complex; hence there are nuances in how one approaches different types of error. Though we cannot go about listing all the different kinds of

---

[3] Singapore Medical Council. 2016. Ethical Code and Ethical Guidelines. Singapore.

medical error known to have occurred, there are some general different types that we should attempt to differentiate:

1) Procedural complications can occur in the best hands, which is why discussion of potential risks as part of informed consent is ethico-legally mandatory. occurs, which is a known risk of a procedure. They remain distressing and when they do occur we must disclose these adverse events to patients and support them to the best of our abilities. Additionally, those of us who are procedurists should do our diligent best to gain experience and drive down complication rates, and have the wisdom to know when to seek help should a particular patient or procedure goes beyond our level of expertise.
2) Drug side effects can be severe and unanticipated (e.g., Stevens Johnson syndrome to an antibiotic). Similar to (1), these are not always avoidable and our duty becomes disclosure and harm mitigation.
3) Frank error resulting in patient harm, such as a wrong-site surgery, a missed critical laboratory result, or medication error such as incorrect insulin administration in a 10ml syringe (10ml = 1000 units) instead of an insulin syringe (10 markings = 10 units). Such errors are serious, can lead to claims of medical

negligence, yet can happen to any of us especially if tired or overloaded.

4) Suboptimal management resulting in patient harm, for instance delayed recognition of a medically deteriorating patient, or the lack of medical knowledge resulting in a patient not receiving the best treatment. This is often due to a skill or knowledge deficit, which will demand that we as junior doctors make the utmost effort to overcome as we grow in our medical careers. In this, continuing medical education to improve our patient care is not only a professional imperative, but also an ethical and spiritual one, that we may become better stewards of patient lives.

5) Willful negligence, where a doctor blatantly and deliberately ignores his or her responsibilities or causes patient harm. This should not happen at all.

Regardless of the type of medical error, several scriptural principles guide us.

We are fallible

A repeated but oft forgotten truth that the Bible tells all Christians is that we are fallible. We have all sinned and fallen short of the glory of God (Romans 3:23). We are tempted to laziness and sloth, therefore we are tempted to cut corners. We, like Jesus' disciples are also weak in the flesh

(Matthew 26:41), hence we fall asleep, have our judgement impaired, and make mistakes in our work.

As doctors we might be resistant to admitting this truth. We might be tempted to believe that some unspecified amount of hard work can bring us close enough to perfection, such that we might one day never again make a mistake. This belief is foolish and unbiblical because it goes against Scripture that tell us we are imperfect and will never be able to make ourselves perfect through human means. Scripture calls us to recognise our imperfection even as we lean on the Holy Spirit to guide and empower all the work we do.

We are not fully in control

Additionally, us doctors need to realise that God is the one in control, not us. Paul writes in 1 Corinthians 3:7

> *"So neither the one who plants nor the one who waters is anything, but only God, who makes things grow."*

Paul is using a farming analogy to represent how labourers (such as himself and Apollo) in Christian ministry are merely instruments playing their part to plant seeds of faith and water the faith of the new church. God, however, is the only one who can actually make these people grow. In the same way, while we Christian doctors are the ones who are given the privilege of wielding the knowledge and the instruments of healing, we are *not* the ones ultimately in control. God brings about healing in the same way he makes the plants grow: by His power and His grace. We are merely vessels of His, like the farmers who plants the seeds or waters the plants.

Therefore, we do not have full control over what happens to our patients or how they respond. We are given the weighty burden of using our skills and knowledge to the best of our ability. But we must recognise that the results are not guaranteed because we cannot always control the outcome completely or predict all possibilities. God can give and God can take away, so we cannot operate daily on the basis that our patients remain alive solely through our human effort and intellect. Instead, we are called to give our absolute best by stewarding our gifts well, realising that the true fate of our patients lies in the hands of God.

To a certain extent, the medical world has come to recognise that no one doctor, nurse, or therapist is likely to be the sole person responsible for patient safety. The "Swiss Cheese Model" depicts that errors are often not the consequence of a single point of failure or one individual's mistake, instead, multiple vulnerabilities ("holes in the cheese") need to line up for patient harm to occur. Therefore, if we are faced with a situation that has resulted in patient harm, we should not be too quick to blame only ourselves, but instead realise that there might not be a single person to bear all the blame alone. However, as doctors, we play a central role in patient care and therefore still bear significant responsibility for their harm.

Response to making a Medical Error

All that being said, we cannot stop there. It is woefully insufficient to claim that mistakes were made because we are fallible and because we are not totally in control. The calling to Christians in the medical profession is centred around loving our patients and doing the best for them. When a doctor makes a mistake and harms a patient, this calling remains the same. Even after committing a medical error, we are still called to love them in whatever way possible, even at significant cost to ourselves.

Truth and Integrity

If a medical error is made, we Christians are called to be people of integrity and truth (Proverbs 12:22). Unfortunately there have been instances of physicians attempting to cover up, shift blame to others, or even retrospectively amend medical records. But open disclosure is not only a requirement of the Singapore Medical Council's ethical code, it is in line with obedience to Christ in trying to love our patients sacrificially, putting their welfare first, and preventing further errors from occurring. Practically, this is not a task that junior doctor should take on themselves, but one that should be escalated in line with hospital policy. What our gospel calls us to do may seem foolish to those who prize their career and reputation above all. But we are called to live by God's standards and not the world's.

Genuine Correction

While medical error is not the same as committing a sin, there is a similar brokenness in how it causes harm to God's creation. Hence, we are called to make sincere attempts to mitigate the harm caused, and make sure that we right the wrong where we can. This may include detailed explanations about the issue, closer monitoring after an incident, appropriate treatment for ensuing complications, and so on. The underlying principle here is that we are not meant to run away from our wrongdoing nor hide from a neighbour whom we have hurt. We should put our best foot forward to love that neighbour and ensure that they get the treatment that they need.

We can also pray for the patients that we have hurt. They are humans too under God's sovereign will. Praying for them and for God to deliver them is entirely biblical, and helps our hearts be attuned to their needs and their pain. We can pray for God to protect them from the mistake caused by our own hands. If the damage has already been done, we can pray that God the true healer will bring them healing.

The Call to Excellence

Finally, any medical error (or a healthy fear of medical error) should remind us of our call to be excellent. The sanctity of all human life created in the image of God Himself should drive us to treat the well-being of our patients with reverent awe, and to work as unto the Lord (Colossians 3:22). It is easy to become complacent or do 'just enough' when patient care becomes routine or when clinical demands are heavy. But honouring God with our work *and* remembering the sanctity of the lives placed under our care should mean that we take extra care to make sure that every history and examination is excellent, every counselling session is done properly, and every procedure is done to our utmost ability. Yet there is a distinction between doing so from a sincere desire to do our work excellently, rather than the crippling anxiety of causing harm.

Additionally an attitude of excellence towards building our medical knowledge and skills protects our future patients and glorifies God in our work. This does not mean that our work is flawless from the get-go, nor does it mean that we are called to be neurotic and obsessive. It does, however, mean that our work is the best we can do and filled with integrity and compassion for God's children. If it requires us to put in extra hours at work, going the extra mile to educate families, or to be extra careful in our examinations, then we should be doing just that. This can even translate to us spending more time reading up on conditions we are unfamiliar with, or voicing out our weaknesses when we know we may short-change a patient.

Guilt and Shame

Many physicians report feelings of guilt and shame as a result of medical error. Satan is the accuser (Revelation 12:10–12), and will no doubt use such a situation to challenge us about our calling and our desire to do God's work in the medical field. Whether or not we receive forgiveness from the patient or their family, we receive grace and forgiveness from God if we are repentant and humble in heart. While sorrow is natural and right, we cannot let guilt and shame overwhelm us to the point of harming ourselves or walking away from what God has called us to do. For our work has been redeemed by Jesus' greater work on the cross. We are called to toil with the expectant hope that Jesus will one day return, and the new creation will come. Revelation 21:4 promises us that He will wipe away every tear, that there will be no more crying or pain, and death shall be no more. We need to hold on to that promise.

Leaning on community

Though easy to say, it is extremely difficult to have the right frame of mind when facing such a scenario. Even armed with knowledge, we are likely to struggle when we encounter this. Navigating the aftermath of a medical error thus necessitates the support of a Christian community. We should seek out seniors who have faced similar situations themselves, and whom you can process these thoughts together with. In all likelihood, your seniors and mentors in medicine have encountered such scenarios before and will have something to offer. Even if their experience is not directly relatable to your current one, they can and should walk with you through this. As the Bible says, we should weep with those who weep (Romans 12:15).

We are called to turn to community and to turn to Jesus when we feel like we have failed (more in the next chapter). This is because we were never created to walk this path alone, nor are we called to grapple with our calling as a lone wolf.

Discussion questions:

1. Reflect on the concept of human fallibility. How does acknowledging our fallibility help us deal with the pressures and challenges of professional life in the medical field?

2. How can we contribute to the healing process for both patients (and family) and healthcare professionals when errors are made?

3. How can we balance the call for excellence in our work with the understanding of our limitations as humans?

4. How can we effectively support our peers and colleagues who may be struggling with guilt and shame after making a mistake at work?

WHEN WE FAIL – DEALING WITH DEFEAT

Sarah felt like an absolute failure. This was the sixth month of being a doctor, yet she could not even grasp the basics. She struggled to do "simple things" like memorising her patient's input and output amounts, knowing how to respond to common medical emergencies, and remembering all the tasks she needed to do. Every week since starting work, she had gotten scolded by seniors, screamed at by patients' family members, or had some mistake be rectified by other doctors or nurses. She feels that she has only gotten this far due to the help she has received from her fellow colleagues. As she walks out of the hospital, her friendly ward nurses shout "Bye Doctor Sarah! See you tomorrow!". Sarah waves back and smiles, but deep down she knows she does not deserve the title of 'Doctor'. Deep down she feels like an absolute imposter because she just cannot seem to get it right.

Some of us know this feeling. We feel like imposters in our roles as doctors and the repeated failures we have experienced stand as cold, hard evidence that we are not good enough. We feel pressure to be good at our work, to be successful in our careers, yet we somehow cannot figure out how to become the "doctor we are meant to be".

The pressure to be successful

One of the worst things about being a doctor is that the general public often expects us to be perfect. Sarah's sense of imposter syndrome is prevalent amongst our community. Somehow, we doctors are put on a pedestal and not really allowed to fail or make mistakes. We are given a lot of respect and with that comes a tremendous amount of responsibility. This translates into our careers as well, as we spend an ungodly amount of time working, studying, and practising in order to advance at work or pass our exams. This can be really unhealthy and can lead us into an endless chase for more and more success.

The ugly flipside to the success addiction is that once we inevitably fail at something, we internalize the failure and start to associate it with our identity. Instead of thinking, "I failed at this task", we start to think "I am a failure" or some variation of "I am not good enough". Because we exist in a sea of driven, intelligent, and capable individuals, we feel the pressure to keep up and perform at the highest level all the time.

The truth is that how we perceive failure depends a lot on how we view success. If we keep pressuring ourselves to be as successful as the world expects or as our colleagues seem to be, then we have this false idea of success that was put in place by the world. Many times, we chase these ideals without first asking God what He has purposed us to do. We may have been endlessly swept along since we were teenagers, and therefore have not even decided for ourselves what we want to pursue.

Yes, we are called to be excellent at work and to glorify God. But excellence at work does not equate to becoming a senior consultant or the Head of Department. It does mean however, that we are called to be the best doctor that we can be regardless of position. It certainly means that we do not take shortcuts or be lazy, and that we will put in the time and effort to ensure that our patients get the best care we can provide.

Turning to God in our failure

Sometimes however, we genuinely do fail. We fail to live up to expectations or to complete a task that was assigned to us. Sometimes, we become negligent, tired, or careless. We let slip something we should not have, and then someone has to bear the consequences of our failure. As a profession that deals with the literal lives and well beings of others, we often focus on perfection and take failure very badly. Many times, this is justified because a decision that results in death or harm can be irreversible. However, this reality translates into a pervasive need for perfection and high-level performance at all times, even when we are exhausted. While this perfectionist attitude can be helpful at times, it can quickly become toxic when failure in any form turns into self-blame and self-loathing. As with so many other issues mentioned in this book, what the world's culture tells us is wrong and dangerous. We need to turn to the Bible to learn what God tells us about human failure, as well as how He deals with them.

Heroes of the faith, but also failures

Many heroes of the faith in the Bible have been failures. Abraham feared death so he let a king take his wife in marriage. Moses committed murder then had to run for his life. David committed adultery and then tried to cover it up with murder. When we inspect the Bible closely, we realise that all the prominent servants of God were imperfect, and many had grave failures in their time in ministry. However, perhaps the most detailed account of a failure in the Bible is the Apostle Peter. He was one of the first disciples of Jesus, belonged in His inner circle, the first leader of the early church, and an utter failure at the crucial moment.

Peter was clearly highly regarded in the early church. However, the gospel accounts do not try to paint a rosy picture of his rise to power and influence. Instead, these widely distributed accounts take great care to outline the fact that Peter "disowned" Jesus by denying Him. The famous triple denial of Jesus by arguably His most loyal follower should clue us into the fact that all four gospel writers (and God Himself) want us to know how it is like to fail and how to come back to Jesus in repentance.

Peter: The Failure

The story of Peter's denial of Jesus starts before Jesus was even captured. While having the last supper, Jesus predicts that the disciples will "fall away" from him (Matthew 26:31). Upon hearing this, Peter insisted that "even if all fall away on account of you, I never will" (Matthew 26:33). This shows Peters confidence in himself and in his own faith. He has followed Jesus for three years, been at His side through triumph and persecution, and now felt confident that he will not fail Him. Even when Jesus predicts that Peter specifically will disown Him three times by the next morning, Peter declares again that even if he has to die, he will not disown Jesus (Matthew 26:35).

Perhaps some of us can identify with the confidence that Peter had in himself. We junior doctors have been trained for many years and have managed to graduate from medical school. That in itself rightly should be a source of pride and confidence in our own abilities. Furthermore, many of us have spent years in school performing at a high level and often being the cream of the crop. We are like Peter in the sense that we had a good track record and had reasons to be confident or proud.

However, we know that Peter later fails to live up to his promises. All four gospels recount the denials, but Matthew 26:69–75 gives us the most vivid picture of what happened:

"Now Peter was sitting out in the courtyard, and a servant girl came to him. 'You also were with Jesus of Galilee,' she said. But he denied it before them all. 'I don't know what you're talking about,' he said. Then he went out to the gateway, where another servant girl saw him and said to the people there, 'This fellow was with Jesus of Nazareth.' He denied it again, with an oath: 'I don't know the man!'

After a little while, those standing there went up to Peter and said, 'Surely you are one of them; your accent gives you away.' Then he began to call down curses, and he swore to them, 'I don't know the man!'

Immediately a rooster crowed. Then Peter remembered the word Jesus had spoken: 'Before the rooster crows, you will disown me three times.' And he went outside and wept bitterly."

This passage comes as a swift fulfilment of Jesus' prediction. So confident just hours before this denial, Peter now goes outside to weep after cursing and swearing oaths that he does not know Jesus.

All of us can identify with Peter at this point. Instead of disowning Jesus, maybe we made a mistake and that caused harm or death to a patient. Maybe we had high expectations of our performance at work, but we just could not cope and buckled under the pressure. Perhaps we failed to get into our residency of choice after trying for years, or we got into that residency but failed to pass our exams. Whatever the cause, we all experience disappointment, and we have at some point felt like an absolute failure. Some of us might be extremely successful at work but fail outside of it. Many doctors let work so consume us that we neglect our families, friends, faith, or even our spouse. Perhaps while immersed in this rigorous and toxic culture, we have abandoned our life and faith at the door to the hospital. No matter the cause, our failures are painful and crippling. It can feel like our lives are over and we have nothing left, so we weep as Peter did.

Whatever the case, Jesus calls us back from the brink. Remember that Jesus came not to call the righteous, but sinners (Mark 2:17). He came to fellowship with the failures and the ostracized of this world, not the proud and the "perfect".

Peter is forgiven

Peter's redemption comes at the hands of the resurrected Jesus. After Jesus rose from the dead, He went to meet His disciples. At this point, the disciples were still a bunch of scared, defeated men. They went back to their old profession before they followed Jesus, which was to fish. John 21 gives a detailed account of this episode. When Peter (still on the boat) realises that it is Jesus on the shore, he jumps out of the boat and swims to Him as fast as he can. When he finally gets to talk to Jesus, they have this strange but deeply meaningful conversation. This conversation is most commonly titled "Jesus Reinstates Peter", meaning that Peter is restored and forgiven by Jesus.

John 21:15–19 – Jesus Reinstates Peter

"When they had finished eating, Jesus said to Simon Peter, 'Simon son of John, do you love me more than these?'

'Yes, Lord,' he said, 'you know that I love you.'

Jesus said, 'Feed my lambs.'

Again, Jesus said, 'Simon son of John, do you love me?'

He answered, 'Yes, Lord, you know that I love you.'

Jesus said, 'Take care of my sheep.'

The third time he said to him, 'Simon son of John, do you love me?'

Peter was hurt because Jesus asked him the third time, 'Do you love me?' He said, 'Lord, you know all things; you know that I love you.'

Jesus said, 'Feed my sheep.

Very truly I tell you, when you were younger you dressed yourself and went where you wanted; but when you are old you will stretch out your hands, and someone else will dress you and lead you where you do not want to go.' Jesus said this to indicate the kind of death by which Peter would glorify God. Then he said to him, 'Follow me!'"

Through the repeated questioning of Peter, Jesus was leading him through the process of repentance, and in that process also giving him the greatest calling he would ever receive. Earlier in the gospel story, Jesus tells Peter that upon this rock (Peter), He will build His church (Matthew 16:18). Now, He reaffirms this statement and tells Peter to "feed [His] lambs". This is a commission to nurture and to grow the church of Jesus Christ. To use his experience (both triumphs and failures) to feed and strengthen his brothers and sisters in Christ.

In Peter's whole redemption arc, there 3 denials, 3 questions of "do you love me?" and 3 instructions of "feed my lambs".

The number "3" is very significant in the Bible. It is often used to symbolize completeness and absoluteness (e.g. the Holy Trinity; or when God is described as 'Holy, Holy, Holy; or when Jesus rose on the 3rd day to conquer death). With the reinstatement of Peter, this number holds clear meaning from start to end as well. The 3 initial denials represent complete abandonment of Jesus in the face of danger, signaling that Peter truly failed his master – contrary to his bold promises. Once reunited after the resurrection, the 3 times that Jesus asked "Peter do you love me" and the three times that Peter said "Yes I do love you" represents the complete repentance on Peter's part for his betrayal. Finally, the three times that Jesus insists "feed my lambs" represents the absolute command and special commission of Jesus to Peter, tasking him with the responsibility of growing and guiding the church. Peter will go on to serve faithfully for his whole life, even after Jesus predicts that he will suffer and die for this cause (John 21:18–19).

How should we react to failure?

Though we all fail differently and face different struggles, reading this account of Peter's failure gives us some critical learning points. Most of us naturally react in despair or tears at first—this is normal. However, we need to start turning to God as the only true source of help.

Turning to your fellow Christians

Pastor Rick Warren of Saddleback church made an interesting observation in one of his sermons on the disciples' reactions just after the crucifixion of Jesus. Having seen the death of their beloved Saviour and their only source of hope (as they had left everything to follow Him), they were shaken to the core. We know that Peter in particular was severely affected by his own denial of Jesus. However, when the disciples are mentioned in the immediate period after Jesus died, they are always gathered together. Mark 16:10 mentions how Mary went to their house but found them "together grieving and weeping". They were scared of the Jewish leaders and so stuck together behind locked doors (John 20:19).

The Bible gives us an explicit command in Galatians 6:2 to "bear one another's burdens", stating that by doing this we fulfil the law of Christ. In talking about love for one another, Paul instructs us to "weep with those who weep" (Romans 12:15). This is clear indication for us as Christians to be there for one another especially when we encounter catastrophic failures in our lives. We don't need to have solutions, nor do we need to know what to say. As a first step, we just need to turn to each other and weep together, encouraging each other to look to Christ. It is not always easy to have trustworthy friends, family, or Christian accountability partners in the workplace whom we can turn to in such times. This is why we should try to actively build and maintain godly relationships with others who can bear our burdens with us, even when we are busy at work.

Turn to Jesus in desperation

When Peter sees Jesus from the boat in John 21, he immediately jumps off the boat and swims towards Him. He cannot even wait for the boat to sail to shore. He is so desperate to come back to his Lord, seeking reconciliation in light of his massive failure. Like Peter, we too are in desperate need of Jesus, especially when we feel like a failure. Though it is not likely that we find ourselves in a similar situation like Peter's to reject Jesus, we often slowly turn our backs on Him over time when we lose sight of Him in this life.

In these situations, God calls us to turn back to Him. We can turn to God because His character is consistent throughout the whole Bible: slow to anger, quick to forgive, and abounding in love. Lamentations 3:22–23 reminds us that the steadfast love of the Lord never ceases, and that His mercies are new every morning. 2 Timothy 2:13 similarly tells us that even if we are faithless, God remains faithful to us. We even know that Jesus prays and intercedes on our behalf (Hebrews 7:25 and Romans 8:34). Hence, we will do well to put away our old self, the one that is always anxious to succeed and keeps striving in order to earn favour. We need to put on this new self, the one who knows that God loved us even when we were still sinners. Remember that God loves us not because we are so lovable, but because it is in His nature. God is also our comforter in all our troubles (2 Corinthians 1:3), and He invites us to turn to Him.

This is why Peter desperately jumped out of the boat to get to Jesus. He could not wait to go back to His Lord and repent of his failure. We can do the same, and we know that we will be met with forgiveness.

We are called to use our failures to strengthen others

Luke's gospel provides us with another account of Jesus' prediction of Peter's failure. In Luke 22:31–32, Jesus says:

"Simon, Simon, Satan has asked to sift each of you like wheat. But I have pleaded in prayer for you, Simon, that your faith should not fail. So when you have repented and turned to me again, strengthen your brothers.'"

Here we see that Jesus predicts the struggles of the disciples using the analogy of "sifting" by Satan. This separation of wheat from the chaff is a clear image of severe testing, in which the disciples ultimately failed by running away. Jesus knows that Peter and the disciples will fail and instructs him to "strengthen [his] brothers" once he has repented and turned back to Jesus. This echoes the command of Jesus to Peter to "feed [his] lambs".

Peter goes on to do amazing things in his career as the early church's first leader. Soon after Jesus ascends to heaven, he gives the sermon at Pentecost, during which the Holy Spirit of God descends upon all the believers gathered. Now redeemed from his initial cowardice, Peter spends the rest of his life preaching boldly about the good news of Jesus, despite persecution from Jewish authorities. Besides growing the church in Jerusalem, he writes letters (1 Peter and 2 Peter) to encourage believers till this day. Clearly, his experience with Jesus gave him a glimpse of God's mercy and provision, teachings he passes on to the Christians in his letters. Peter the church leader did not ask the gospel writers to omit his utterly embarrassing backstory. Instead, it has stood as a testament to God's mercy and a reminder that God's strength is made perfect in our weaknesses (2 Corinthians 12:9).

We can and should do the same. As we rise in seniority in the medical field, our mistakes and failures need not be shackles that bind us. Instead, they can be displayed for others to see so that others are helped, and God is glorified through us.

In summary, we can see that God continues to build His church and accomplish His purposes no matter how much we fail. In fact, the foundational truth of our entire faith is in an apparent failure (the death of our Messiah) that was redeemed by God (the resurrection of that Messiah). Jesus Christ built His church upon Peter who was redeemed and reinstated by Him. Therefore, God can and will continue to use our failures to accomplish His perfect will on this earth. We just need to trust in Him and come to Him when we fall. As John Piper famously said in his podcast 'Ask Pastor John' on the episode titled 'Reckoning with Personal Failure': "*The evidence of being a Christian is not that there are no tactical defeats in the war, but that you keep fighting till the promised victory is given.*"

Discussion Questions:

1. Have you ever felt pressure from society or your family to perform or be perfect? How does this manifest in your life?

2. When have you felt like a failure in your professional or personal life? Share your experience and how it affected your self-perception.

3. Explore examples of biblical figures who faced failure, such as Abraham, Moses, and David. How did their failures shape their journeys of faith, and what can we learn from them?

4. How can we use our individual failures to encourage and strengthen others? How can God use these failures for His glory?

WHEN WE BECOME CYNICAL – NEGATIVITY IN OUR HEARTS

Emma was once an idealistic and compassionate doctor who entered surgical residency with a heart full of hope. However, the relentless work hours and the unyielding nature of the healthcare system began to chip away at her optimism. The weight of disappointments and the daily struggles with an overloaded system took their toll on Emma's spirit. Slowly, the negativity that festered at work seeped into every facet of her life. Emma's once warm and caring demeanour turned cold, affecting her relationships with her parents, husband, and children. Emma's words, laced with bitterness, became hurtful arrows that pierced the hearts of her loved ones. Even at home, Emma couldn't escape the weight of her cynicism. Her interactions with her spouse became strained, and her children felt the sting of their mother's biting remarks. The once vibrant household echoed with the silence of resentment.

The work culture in this day and age is rife with negativity. Since the start of medical school, many students are bombarded with messages that are predominantly negative.

Students shadow junior doctors and are told things like "quit while you still can", or to "open your eyes and see what a horrible life this is". Social media expose many negative accounts of working in the healthcare system, as well as systemic issues that plague the workplace. Many junior doctors emphasize the struggles they face at work while speaking to their juniors, such as long hours, abuse from patients and their families, and workplace politics and struggles. And rightly so! These are serious issues that need to be worked through and should not be left status quo. Many of these are truthful and often not isolated events. It is in fact a good thing that the struggles and abuses of healthcare workers has been brought to light in the public space in recent times, to encourage more honest conversations and resolution with decisive measures by policymakers that may not otherwise know of issues on the ground.

However, we ought to be careful of the detrimental side effects of this culture: negativity, gossip, and jadedness. Many find solace and refuge in complaining about work, vilifying co-workers or superiors who they perceive as having done them wrong, and in some sense, boasting about how terrible their life is. Perhaps this is a coping mechanism for many of us and we cannot help but find some comfort in the complaining. Maybe this 'trend' has gotten to us because so many of our friends have taken on this attitude, and it is natural to want to be a part of the conversation and share common experiences with colleagues whom we spend so much time with. However, we should be wary of all this negativity and gossip, lest we find ourselves like Emma above, for it is not healthy for us and certainly not the way to act as God's representatives in the workplace.

As we turn to Scripture, we can take comfort in the fact that these feelings are only natural for humans. In Galatians 5:19–20, Paul writes that the "acts of the flesh" include things such as hatred, discord, jealousy, and envy. All of us can identify with these feelings at some point in time. After all, we are only human too. However, if we allow these to take hold in our lives, then we arrive at a general spirit of negativity towards the world and life in general. This is understandable for those who do not have Christ in their lives, because this world on its own is truly hopeless and passing away (1 John 2:17). We as believers in Jesus are different, called to be set aside from the world. As mentioned in the earlier chapter, Christ has redeemed our world and our work. We have been given a new purpose to work and a new purpose to live!

Why we should avoid negativity

Complaining is a genuinely easy and often comforting coping mechanism for all of us. However, it has the dangerous side effect of bringing out rage and fuelling lasting anger and ungodly thoughts in us. When we as Christians spend a lot of our time complaining about work, it will start to cloud out the truly good and God-glorifying aspects of our work. It prevents us from seeing God's hand in the blessing of others through us as vessels and makes us focus on the toiling and fruitless aspect of work.

Being a Christian therefore involves having been redeemed and seeing hope from God's perspective. All of us who accept Jesus Christ as our Lord and Saviour have the Holy Spirit to guide in how we live. Immediately after Paul writes about the "acts of the flesh" (Galatians 5:19–20), he directly contrasts it with the fruit of the Spirit. Some of us are familiar with it: love, joy, peace, forbearance, kindness, goodness, faithfulness, gentleness, and self-control (Galatians 5:22–23). These are fruit that we will bear if we allow the Spirit to work in us in the journey of sanctification. If we are fall into the trap of negativity and complaining, we join in the hostility, pride, and complaining that marks a non-believer who has no hope in Christ for the redemption of this world.

A slippery slope

Have you ever noticed how, once we are annoyed, everything else is suddenly so much more irritating? When something pisses us off in the morning before work, every red light, every spilt drink, and every minor inconvenience is suddenly infuriating. This might be the case for many of us regarding our medical work. When we start to adopt an unnecessarily critical and antagonistic attitude towards our workplace, every single thing we encounter becomes something negative that fuels and compounds our original hatred.

This reinforces our detrimental attitude at work and causes us to dishonour God and harm other people. A nurse might be doing a good job in obeying genuinely good protocol and pointing out your mistake so you don't get into trouble. However, in your annoyance you raise your voice at her. A pharmacist might spot your medication error, saving a patient's life and preventing you from committing a serious reportable fault at work. But you are angry because now you have to log in to the computer again and change your original prescription. Your boss might point out valid and good learning points which will help you be a better doctor in the future. But you become resentful because he might have made you look bad in front of other people.

If we let ourselves start down this slippery slope of constant negativity, we might soon find ourselves in an unbridled descent into a blackhole of negative thoughts that does not just affect ourselves but everyone around us.

Affecting your loved ones and yourself

Like many other destructive behaviours, uncontrolled negativity will be highly detrimental to yourself. Even if we ignore the loss of potential work relationships, we still have to realise that we harm ourselves by bring down our own mental well-being.

If we allow unbridled negativity to pervade throughout our work life, it is likely to bleed into any other situation given enough time. We form habits by what we repeatedly do. Hence, we learn to habitually identify the negative things about any situation that we face, work related or otherwise. This tends to crowd out the positive aspect and makes us lose the joy of being at work. There may come a time when helping to cure a patient's severe illness or being a decisive factor in the life-saving process does not even stir our hearts to joy anymore because we are addicted to focusing on the negative aspects. We might successfully pick up a deteriorating patient on call and save his life with decisive treatment and might even get recognised for it; yet find no joy in such a precious accomplishment of a life saved because we focus on the fact that we didn't get much sleep that night. We might finally get into our residency of choice and yet become very anxious because we realise that more work awaits us in the coming years.

This voluntary but initially imperceptible shift in attitude can start to take a serious toll on our mental health. We might start to become nihilistic and aimless both at work and outside of work. We might start to become depressed with constant self-inflicted low moods. This often leads us to making decisions out of spite or for escapism rather than truly weighing the options properly. Even when we take leave for a long holiday or have an enjoyable time over the weekend, we immediately become depressed when it is over because we dread coming back to the workplace (e.g., having Monday blues or post-leave blues).

Even worse, we might bring this depressive mood home to our families. Our spouses, parents, siblings, and even children will be affected when we come home sad or angry. They will face the brunt of our rage, snide remarks, or our sadness, because they are the ones who greet us at the door when we come home. It does not take a medical degree to know that spending time with a nihilistic, sarcastic, and pessimistic individual can make us more unhappy. How much more so if this person is a spouse, parent, or child? Simple conversations can become an argument because of high irritability, joyful accomplishments at work or school get brushed off because we are "not in the mood to talk about this now". If we think about it, most of our relationships are developed in these small, precious, seemingly inconsequential moments, but we miss or waste these moments if we perpetually and willingly allow negativity and jadedness to bleed into our homes.

Speaking truth in love

No matter which career path you choose to take in medicine, you will grow in seniority and influence. You will inevitably influence some co-workers as you share your experience and dish out advice to medical students who come under your wing. People will listen to what you have to say because it matters, and many will internalize it. This is a solemn and important truth all of us need to understand and grapple with. This is why we as Christian doctors who grow in maturity in the workplace need to learn to speak the truth in love (Ephesians 4:15).

Speaking the truth in this case is easy. Many who speak negatively and gossip about others are often telling the truth! But love for one another is how we are to be known as Jesus' disciples (John 13:34–35) and speaking in a way that is loving is a truly challenging prospect. Luckily, an easy guiding principle on understanding how to be loving is found in 1 Corinthians 13:4–7, otherwise known as "the love passage":

Love is patient, love is kind. It does not envy, it does not boast, it is not proud. It does not dishonor others, it is not self-seeking, it is not easily angered, it keeps no record of wrongs. Love does not delight in evil but rejoices with the truth. It always protects, always trusts, always hopes, always perseveres.

This is simple to say, but really hard to achieve. However, this should not stop us from trying to pursue this behaviour in favour of the easy but dishonouring patterns of negativity. It takes continuing grace from God, and we need to rely on the Holy Spirit to guide us to become more and more Christ-like each day.

The inconvenient reality is that the situation in our hospitals is not ideal. The work demands can be extremely strenuous and often unsustainable. People sometimes are mean, and life is genuinely tough. Legitimate complaints from junior doctors are sometimes not heard by higher ups, or they are heard but seemingly ignored. We should not falsely cover up these faults and declare to the world that 'all is good and we are coping well'.

We as children of God should not lie and cover up too, because that also is not speaking the truth in love. Instead, we can boldly speak the truth in ways that are constructive and push towards genuine solutions and impetus for change. We can build up and bless others with our words and tear down constructively yet gently at the same time (where appropriate), all while denying our human tendency to complain, badmouth, and cast blame.

Discussion questions:

1. Can you relate to Emma's experience of entering medicine with high hopes and ideals, only to have it whittled down over time and grow cynical? Share a personal experience if applicable.

2. In what ways have you observed or experienced the impact of negative messages and attitudes at work?

3. How does negativity and cynicism prevent us from recognising God's blessing in our lives and work?

4. Reflect on Ephesians 4:15 and its call to speak the truth in love. How can we as Christian junior doctors balance truth with a spirit of love and grace?

PART 4: MENTAL HEALTH AND WORK

MENTAL HEALTH AND BURNOUT

James was always keen and caring. When he started practising as a junior doctor, he carried that into his work every single day. Fuelled by a strong desire to help, he dived into the demanding environment with unwavering optimism. However, as weeks turned into tiring months, the never-ending tasks began to wear down his spirit. James found himself stuck in a constant whirlwind of sleepless nights and tough shifts. The initial excitement turned into a heavy tiredness, and the once lively doctor felt like a shadow of his former self. The constant demands and emotional weight of patient struggles became a burden too heavy to bear.

Burnout quietly crept into James' life, chipping away at his strength. His dedication crumbled under the weight of exhaustion, affecting not only his work life but also his personal one. Worried friends and family started to notice the change over time. Internally, James battled with the growing pressure, questioning the very heart of his passion for healing. Feelings of loneliness and self-doubt clouded his thoughts, casting shadows on the once bright path he had envisioned.

James' story is familiar to many of us in one form of another. We come into medicine with a strong desire to help other people but over time are worn down by a multitude of factors. Slowly but surely, we burn out and start to falter. We are not alone. Many junior doctors have described themselves to be burnt out, whether presently or at some point in their career. According to the World Health Organization and ICD-11, burn-out[4] is a syndrome conceptualised as a result of chronic workplace stress that has not been successfully managed. It is characterised by three dimensions:

1) Feelings of energy depletion or exhaustion;
2) Increased mental distance from one's job, or feelings of negativism or cynicism related to one's job; and
3) Reduced professional efficacy.

Without a doubt, burnout is something that has been present in the workplace long before it was a buzz topic amongst millennials and Gen Z on social media. However, people who openly admit to suffering from it had always been heavily stigmatised and even silenced or belittled at the

---

[4] World Health Organization. Burn-out an "occupational phenomenon": International Classification of Diseases.

workplace. In the medical field, it might be easier to see why many accomplished and senior doctors will do this to their fellow colleagues. What is surprising is that this stigma also exists in our churches and Christian circles. We have somehow mistakenly allowed ourselves to think that people who 'follow God's will' or who 'are passionate about their work' or who have 'a clear calling' will never falter or not experience burnout or other mental illnesses. This phenomenon is not remotely limited to the Christians in the medical field. It includes our attitudes towards pastors, ministry workers (e.g., missionaries), and teachers (amongst many others)[5]. If we are to combat it, we need to start making the topic less taboo and allow for frank discussion both in medical circles and in Christian circles.

How the medical field exacerbates burnout

Perhaps one of the ways we can start is by understanding how the medical field exacerbates burnout in both medical students and doctors. First and foremost, the very characteristics of the healthcare environment puts clinicians at a relatively high risk of burnout. Time pressure, lack of control over work processes, and role conflict make most

---

[5] Beavis WJ. Precipitating factors that lead to stress and burnout in restoration movement church pastors: A qualitative study (Doctoral dissertation, The Chicago School of Professional Psychology).

workdays stressful. Furthermore, the lack of control over leave and vacations provide uncertainty in our personal lives. These, combined with the emotional intensity of clinical work already predispose us to burnout.

Another sizeable contributor to burnout is the excessive workload we undertake when we work in medicine. It is no secret that our workload is very high. But on top of that, we need to endure sleep deprivation, long nights, weekend work, and work overtime without compensation. What adds to the hopelessness previously mentioned is the very real possibility that our work hours might not decrease as we become more senior in the workplace. This high workload is viewed as a given in the medical field, and sometimes does not even make allowances for personal circumstance such as family commitments, personal adverse events, or health struggles. This can make it seem like we are very much alone in facing these issues or force us into a corner where quitting becomes the only viable option.

Deeper than these, however, are undercurrents in the workplace that we need to confront and take corrective action if we are to start overcoming these issues in the profession.

Culture of striving

First of all, the culture of medicine is highly competitive. Every year, many students compete to get into medical school. Following that, those that get into medical school strive very hard to do well academically, gain valuable experience, gain favour from bosses in their rotations, and make connections in their desired field. Once they graduate, they compete to get into their desired residency of choice. If successful, they have to work hard to learn and acquire skills and compete for job opportunities at the tail end of their residency. Even if they get a consultant job, a young associate consultant has to work hard to prove him/herself in the department, and a consultant who leaves for the private sector has to start from scratch to build a patient base.

This competitive and highly demanding culture is pervasive and widespread in the medical field. There sometimes seems to be no possible end in sight to competition and striving. This sense of hopelessness and despair is so often seen in junior doctors today and is a serious contributor to our burnout rates.

As Christian doctors, perhaps one of the most important questions we need to ask ourselves is: What am I striving so hard for? Many of us were brought up to unquestioningly pursue career advancement for the sake of it. Many of us (to varying degrees) have gone along with this path without every truly considering deeply why we commit the vast majority of our time and effort into the pursuit of a better job. We tend to default to the answer that "God wants us to be excellent at our work". While that is true, excellence does not equate to grinding till we become Head of Department (HOD) for General Surgery or the CEO of a hospital. It does however mean that we work with absolute integrity, have compassion on our peers and patients, and never take shortcuts with our work no matter who is watching us. Let us not conflate our capitalist ideologies of perpetual striving for vague notions of economic advancement with our Christian calling to true work excellence.

Rather, we should ask God daily what He wants us to accomplish in our workplace, then pursue that calling excellently. Some of us might indeed be called to become the HOD of General Surgery, but others might be called simply to bless others by being a meticulous and excellent resident physician of a hospital. Some of us might not know our end point but are called to do our best to love God and love others in our assigned workplace each day. Whichever the case, our culture needs to change from striving for career advancement to striving toward where God calls us to be. Striving for God and with the Holy Spirit as our helper not only prevents burnout (a rather low bar to set) but gives us the fuel to burn strong and steady for the glory of God no matter where we are placed.

Silence

Silence around these types of issues can severely work against us as well. Many of us have subconsciously (or consciously) attributed mental health struggle to weakness. We fear to voice out the fact that we are struggling because we think that others will judge us for being weak or incapable.

Furthermore, many of us have been stellar students all our lives, consistently performing at a high level and rarely facing failures (if at all). All of a sudden, we find ourselves faltering and struggling to even keep our heads above the water. The expectations we have built up for ourselves and the toxic striving of our culture conflate in the worse possible way and confirms our worse fears: we are useless, weak, or stupid. We burn out because we hold ourselves to an impossible standard and then try to live up to it every day. Then we proceed to exacerbate it by keeping silent when we fall short and start to drown. We end up becoming a cesspool of imperfect people who refuse to admit to our imperfections. Many of us also fear the practical implications of uncovering our struggles with burnout and mental health. We fear that if we were to end up being clinically diagnosed with a psychiatric illness such as depression or anxiety, we might cause our future career to suffer. Whatever the reasons, the result is that we surround our struggle with shame and secrecy, and this continues to fester.

Realising our true identity in Christ is the only true way to freedom. Some tend towards the belief that we are merely a part of a bigger whole, and hence believe that we need to keep silent about our issues, keep our heads down, and play our part. Others tends towards self-actualization and autonomy, so it encourages us to think the best of ourselves and love ourselves without changing for the better. The gospel opposes both such views. It shows us that we are more imperfect than we ever dared to believe, and more loved than we ever dared to hope. This grants us the ability to speak openly about our imperfections, our insecurities, our sins, and our inability to "do it all". Yet, we know simultaneously that none of these aforementioned struggles threaten our identity as loved and forgiven children of God. The freedom that this knowledge grants allows us to recognise that yes, we are weak, but we are loved, and we are complete. We do not have to keep the silence around such issues. It is not that we are perfect the way we are and therefore we deserve better treatment. Instead, we freely admit our weaknesses and struggles because God's power is made perfect in our weakness. Somehow, God will use our weakness for His glory.

Consequences of hiding burnout

Harm to self

Keeping silent and hiding signs of burnout can be really harmful to ourselves. The constant pressure we give ourselves coupled with the self-imposed isolation due to shame or fear of stigma does damage us especially in the long term. By hiding it, we are likely to continue to receive no help and will end up descending further into burnout. We put ourselves at risk of developing depression and anxiety, and we sometimes slowly push away the people who really love and care for us. As our mood worsens, we put ourselves in danger of self-harm behaviours (e.g., cutting, substance abuse, or even suicide).

On the work front, we do ourselves no favours either. It might be true that in the short term, hiding our burnout might be beneficial to our workplace advancement. However, in the long term, we make poorer choices, become more jaded, and we do our work more poorly. We treat people worse as well when we are tired and burnt out. This might seriously damage our career if we allow it to continue. If we allow this behaviour to negatively affect work relationships, this will also harm our ability to interact with our colleagues. This often causes the workplace to become a toxic and high-tension environment, bringing further harm to ourselves and our mental health.

Harm to others

Hidden burnout and mental health issues will not just harm the doctor providing the medical care. It will also go on to harm their patients and whoever they interact with at work. Burnt out doctors will be less careful, less likely to detect things, and more prone to mistakes. Even if we manage to detect such mistakes, we might have the tendency to be tardier with our work and purposely not bother to correct mistakes or brush off criticism for our own good.

Furthermore, our families and friends suffer when we are burnt out. They bear the brunt of our moodiness and tiredness when they face us most of the time we are not at work. We harm these precious relationships when we decide not to face up to our struggles with burnout and mental illnesses. We start by trying to protect our dignity but end up sacrificing our people for it.

To exacerbate all this, when a doctor sees burnout or mental illness as a "weakness" or a "character flaw", they themselves are likely to translate those beliefs into their practice. As such, if a patient comes to this doctor with impending or existing mental health conditions, the doctor is more likely to brush it off as trivial or pass judgement on that patient's character. Either way, the patient does not get optimal medical care. This is crucial because when we reach this stage, we start to perpetuate the problem of stigmatization in individuals with mental health struggles. We then become part of the problem, harming those whom we pledged to help.

What can we do?

We cannot change the culture of medicine overnight. By ourselves, we will also not be able to solve the manpower issues that plague our healthcare system nor be able to alleviate our workload. However, we can change a few things for ourselves, and we can start to set in motion some changes in the culture of the people immediately around us.

Recognising and addressing mental health issues

Doctors need to be able to get help before their mental health issues impact their ability to take care of their patients. We need to educate and equip ourselves with the ability to recognise the signs and also be willing to tell our colleagues when we see them struggling with mental health. Ironically, so many junior doctors have become burnt out that the warning signs of burning out have become normalised. We have come to expect low mood and jadedness from our junior doctors. We expect them to be sleep deprived, look haggard, and to have low energy levels at work. We make nihilistic jokes and memes about being burnt out or coping with alcohol that we can start to become numb to these very warning signs. Many of us are even surprised on the odd occasion when we see our colleagues walking around with high levels of energy and a positive attitude. However, we have to realise that what is normal is not necessarily what is right. If an entire country is morbidly obese, it would be madness to shift the BMI scale and say that being obese is now totally healthy. The same is true for burnout.

If we can start to recognise burnout in our friend groups and address it openly without shame or stigmatization, perhaps we can set the tone for the generations after us. Perhaps our juniors who inevitably face hardship at work can be picked up by their seniors (us) and be empowered to seek help when needed.

Building a circle of accountability

Another thing we can start to do in our circles is to recognise that we are fragile and imperfect. We are not all-powerful, and we do falter (more often than we would care to admit). Recognising this is not a sign of defeat or failure, but rather that we are self-aware and humble enough to admit to others that we need help. We can start to normalise seeking help, whether from friends, family, or professionals.

God's Word makes it abundantly clear that there is no such thing as 'lone wolf Christianity'. Our faith cannot be practised in isolation from community, and we are always part of a community of believers. We are called to pray together, learn from each other, be accountable for each other, and to bear one another's burdens (Galatians 6:2). Hence, we need to reflect and ask ourselves honestly if we have neglected being accountable to others. Many enter their first year of medicine and immediately lose contact with their church/cell group because of the rigour of medical work. Often, such individuals are not able to find another Christian accountability group to replace the ones they have lost. This results in a large number of Christian doctors who simply do not have many accountability partners (if at all). These doctors then become the proverbial lone wolf Christian, navigating work life, career, young adulthood, parenthood, finance, and many other challenges all by themselves. This puts them at a much higher risk of burning out simply because they have no support close by, no like-minded group of Christians to help them along and keep them accountable.

We may not be burnt out now, but there may very well come a time that we are. It is not exclusively caused by career problems; there could be many aetiologies of burnout. Burnout can be triggered by having a new child, problems with family members or finance, or really anything that can cause us stress. We have to root ourselves in Christian communities and find solid Christian mentors so that we can receive support and help when we stumble, and also extend help to others when we are doing fine. If we start to plant ourselves in accountability groups and normalise this culture of accountability for Christians in the medical field, perhaps we can gain ground on this stubborn issue.

Walking with those who struggle

Even if we ourselves do not struggle with mental illnesses, it is highly likely that we will find ourselves in a position to help or walk alongside someone who does struggle with mental health issues. In our healthcare system, it is common to come across fellow doctors who express (either explicitly or implicitly) that they are not coping well. Many junior doctors feel trapped and caught in a cycle of endless toil, with no hope or end in sight. With physical, mental, and emotional exhaustion being the norm in our hospitals, it is no wonder that mental illness is widespread. Though we cannot treat and solve everyone's issues, it is helpful to have a proper biblical understanding of the issues and equip ourselves to help as best as we can.

The nature of mental illness is such that it is often a chronic issue, with patterns of relapsing and remitting. The process of helping someone through a mental health struggle is often long drawn and almost always exhausting for those who walk beside them. Sometimes, in our impatience and human imperfection, we can start to forget these truths and end up becoming frustrated with and resentful of those we originally tried to help.

One of the most overlooked factors in mental health is how we understand what it means to "get better". For many who hold the "old school" or "traditional" way of thinking, mental health issues are something to be glossed over, something that individuals "just have to suck it up and deal with". Oftentimes mental health issues may be suppressed or swept under the rug. Even if they seek treatment for mental illness, they might have the expectation that the mental illness be cured completely. This is completely untrue of course, as many people with mental illness such as depression and anxiety take time to recover and are likely to relapse again[6].

The other temptation is to work only towards symptom management or reduction, and to accept that the mental illness is part of the identity of the person from this point onwards. This approach would work only to alleviate the signs and symptoms of the mental illness without addressing the root causes and might even neglect to help the person start on the long journey to recovery.

Perhaps the most helpful way to look at the issue is through the lens of a recovery journey. The oxford dictionary defines recovery as "a return to a normal state of health, mind or strength", or the "action or process of regaining possession or control of something stolen or lost". This is helpful because while we do not unfairly expect the afflicted person to "be cured" instantly, we also do not regard their mental state as something that is irreversible, irreparable, or beyond redemption. Instead, we understand that like the process of sanctification, recovery is a journey that takes place over a period of time, with setbacks and failures along the way.

---

[6] Burcusa SL, Iacono WG. Risk for recurrence in depression. Clinical psychology review. 2007 Dec 1;27(8):959-85.

To quote Matthew Stanford from his book *Grace for the Afflicted*:

"The goal of recovery goes far beyond symptom reduction but aims at equipping the individual to live beyond their illness. The most important thing to remember is that recovery is a process. It takes time, it can be messy, and differs from person to person, but people with mental illness can and do recover."

Protecting our mental Health

Protecting our mental health is truly underrated. For the longest time, the general approach to work was the gung-ho attitude in a hustle culture that revolved around buzzwords like "sleep is for the weak" and "I don't rest when I'm tired; I rest when I'm done". Though one can argue that this attitude is useful in some contexts, it can be very harmful to people who ignore self-care and spiritual nourishment in the pursuit of excellence at work. Those who are sucked into this culture of "win at all costs" or "compete or die" often have unhealthy levels of stress and will (especially in the long term) suffer from many downstream effects.

We have to protect our own mental health too, if we are to glorify God at work. People who get into medicine in the first place are often very Type-A in terms of personality. They are high-achieving, passionate, often perfectionistic, and extremely capable. Often these individuals come from a lifetime of good grades and stellar extra-curricular performance. Being so capable is obviously a blessing, but sometimes can also come at a cost. One of these costs is perhaps never learning how to rest or to protect their own mental health. Even as Christians, individuals might not be able to fully find rest in God, if they even know what it means to do so.

By maxing out on this culture of stretching ourselves to the limit each and every day, we quickly burn ourselves out. We find that we are not able to sustain this level of intensity, rapidly reaching a point where we are angry at the system, disappointed at how terrible we are feeling, and are depressed to even go to work anymore. We lose sight of our passions and end up fantasizing about ways to leave and pursue a life that is perhaps more enjoyable. Sometimes, people even burn out to a point where they engage in self-harm themselves or even commit suicide.

We need to have some fundamental shifts in our mindset and to remember biblical truths if we are to continue serving God in the field of medicine.

Remember that we are dust

Psalm 103:13–16 reads:

> *"As a father has compassion on his children,*
>
> *so the Lord has compassion on those who fear him;*

for he knows how we are formed,

he remembers that we are dust.

The life of mortals is like grass,

they flourish like a flower of the field;

the wind blows over it and it is gone,

and its place remembers it no more."

This psalm is very poignant because it reminds us of the frailty of humans. It compares us to dust or to grass in a field. We exist for a short moment of time then we die, insignificant and unremembered. On its own, it can seem strange that verse 13 starts by saying that God has compassion on us, then proceeds to speak about our fleeting existence. But in the grand scheme of the Bible, the fact that God sent Jesus down to die for our sins should blow our minds. He sacrificed His Son for an insignificant blade of grass! Have you ever sat in a crowd and looked up at someone super important on stage? Imagine yourself at a concert with your favourite star, and he notices you, goes down to you, and talks to you in person. You would be honoured that someone so important bothered to notice you! One person in the crowd. Now imagine that, except that this star is the infinite God of the universe, and you are not one in a crowd of ten thousand, but billions of people that have ever existed. That is our greatest honour—that God would notice us and love us; that He would go to such great lengths to have a relationship with us. That is why knowing that we are dust and grass is such an encouragement.

When we work, we sometimes have the tendency to think that we are better than we actually are. Christian doctors are often well intentioned and want to put in their best work to serve God. But in our pride and in our small human minds, we think that if we do not perform, lives will not be saved, things will not get done, or others might screw up something that we wouldn't have. We might also think that if we take a break from the ward work, or if we don't finish that research write-up, things will not get done and we will let down our colleagues and fail at God's calling for us.

A wise pastor once remarked: "Isn't it great that we aren't in charge of making the universe run? We will do such a poor job. It's such a relief that God is sovereign!" Knowing that we are dust, not gods, should be a huge relief to you and me. It is a relief to know that we do not bear the weight of saving lives on our shoulders, and that we are merely stewards of gifts God has given us. We are responsible for being faithful, for giving our best and not being lazy. However, we are not in charge of saving everyone, nor are we responsible for solving every single medical, psychological, or social problem that our patient might have.

Christopher Ash mentions in his book *Zeal Without Burnout*:

"When you and I surrendered to Jesus as Lord, we did not offer him the services of a divine, or even semi-divine creature to strengthen his kingdom; we offer him the fragile, temporary, mortal, frail life that he has first given to us. That is all we have to offer. God knows that. For he knows our frame; he remembers that we are dust."

Ash is saying God knows that He has enlisted the help of a frail human being into His army. In Psalm 103:13 we see that God has compassion on us and knows that we are dust. He is not spiting us for being frail; He loves us while knowing that we are nothing. The impact that we have on God's Kingdom is miniscule, no matter how big it seems to us humans. And to emphasize the point, that is a good thing, not a bad thing. If we had to perform in order to earn love from God, we would not only be incredibly stressed out, but we would fall so far short.

We would do well to remember that we are first and foremost human and finite. That mindset is important—sometimes burnout can happen because we place this overwhelming burden on ourselves, thinking that we have this awesome responsibility to accomplish a task given to us by God. While it is definitely important to be faithful to our calling, we must not fall into the trap of thinking that God's success is somehow dependent on ours through our striving and hard work. The key here is a healthy balance between excellence in what has been entrusted to us (meaning that we should not be lazy or idle) and having the mindset that we are not that significant. We should remember that we are but dust, insignificant in the passage of time. However, we have been given the honour and favour of participating in God's will and to have a relationship with Him. We have significance because God loves us and invites us to come to Him, not by any means of our work accomplishments.

Understanding rest

Rest is one of those things that many type-A, competitive task-oriented people (such as many doctors) find hard to do well. At any point in time, we always feel like there is something to accomplish, some medical condition to read up on, or some research to be done. Even if we have nothing to do, we might go look for things to do. Something to pad our CV, something to add to our life outside of work, or even ways to do work outside of regular work (volunteering, church ministry, etc). Most of us grew up in an always bustling environment, and so we find it hard to rest completely in God. It might even be true that we are addicted to the amount of activity that surrounds us, and we are wound up so tightly that true quiet and stillness of the soul might scare us more than a lifetime of busyness. While all the things mentioned above aren't bad per se, a perpetual desire to be productive and an addiction to "getting things done" can be incredibly toxic to our spirits.

So, when we burn out, a good question to ask ourselves is: have I been intentionally resting? Have I trusted God enough to leave the matters of my life, work, and His ministry in His hands and answer His call to find rest in Him? Or have I pushed forward in my own strength and exceeded my own limits, resulting in burnout? Have I failed to draw proper boundaries and let my worries about career bleed into my rest times?

We as finite creatures were never designed to keep on working without any rest or sustenance. Remember that the Bible tells us that the Sabbath was created for man and not man for the Sabbath (Mark 2:27). This means that the rest day every week is to ensure that we as humans are able to recharge and recover from the week of work, drawing our strength from resting in God. It implies not just that rest is good, but that rest is in fact necessary for us. God is a God who does not slumber nor sleep, and He watches over us day and night. God has unlimited power and energy, and we do not. Our mistake (as was Adam and Eve's mistake in Genesis 3) is to think that we could be like God, having unlimited energy to keep on working and never resting.

Physical Rest

As mentioned in the previous chapter on depression, we must also understand that physical rest cannot be separated from spiritual rest. The biblical understanding is that the spirit and the body are inextricably linked to each other, and sometimes burnout can happen as a result of taking care of one but neglecting the other. It would be a mistake to think that rest and renewal of our spirits is separate from physical rest and refreshment. Being deficient in either physical or spiritual rest can have negative consequences on us, and lack of physical rest can have negative impacts on our spiritual life. For example, if we are lacking in sleep, it is all the easier to be angry, to be poorly disciplined, and to fall prey to temptation than compared to if we were well rested and refreshed. There is no point trying to squeeze in two hours of quiet time if you have only slept for three hours the previous night, and that insistence on clocking the two hours of quiet time might in fact be contributing to your burnout. Sometimes the most God-honouring thing you can do is to get some sleep, exercise, or eat a nutritious meal. After all, your body is a temple unto God (1 Corinthians 6:19–20) and if the temple is unkempt and largely in disarray, then perhaps putting it in order is the best worship you can give to God in that moment.

Discipline of Rest

Ultimately, we need not only consider resting when we are burning out or have burnt out. It is useful to institute regular times of rest in the same way that we encourage the discipline of regularly doing quiet time with Bible reading and prayer. This can take the form of a Sabbath day, but it does not have to be legalistic. Rather, we must understand that regular rest is a God-designed mechanism of restraint in our lives. In His infinite goodness and wisdom, God gives us the gift of rest as a reminder that we are dependent on Him, and that we can enjoy the fruit of our labours even in the midst of the toil.

We need to set boundaries between work and rest, simply because we were designed by God to need time to stop working. When we are at work, we should be intensely focused, efficient, and excellent to the glory of God. When we are meant to be resting, we should be intentionally exclusive and disciplined with carving out time, and put away all work to allow for relaxation, recuperation, and basking in God's presence.

As with most things, if we do not actively put aside protected time to rest both physically and spiritually, the distractions of this world will quickly fill up that space. Whether it is endless work or endless entertainment, things will slowly creep in. The call system in the hospitals is furthermore extremely detrimental to our ability to find physical rest, and there is no simple solution given the current situation.

However, there are times where we can be resting yet are distracted by social media, entertainment, or other forms of work which we might take home from the hospital. Because of this existing handicap, it is all the more important that we learn the discipline of rest, so that we might burn brightly and continuously, and not burn out.

Discussion questions: Burnout

1.   Have you ever felt burnt out? If yes, what do you think contributed to that burnout?

2.   How does understanding your identity in Christ relate to freedom from shame and secrecy?

3.   Reflect on the importance of spiritual accountability in the Christian faith. How has accountability played a role in your spiritual journey?

4.   In what ways can you help others gain close Christian relationships? How can we support and walk alongside colleagues or friends who are struggling?

5.   What is your understanding of rest? How does this relate to your spiritual life?

6.   Given the challenges of your demanding schedule, how can you ensure that you maintain a discipline of rest?

ANXIOUS FOR NOTHING

Sean woke up for a third time that night. His heart was racing and he was in cold sweat. Everything in his room was normal, but he felt an impending sense of doom. For four months straight, he has been experiencing such episodes of anxiety attacks. Even at work in the hospital, he sometimes feels so anxious that he has to go to the toilet to recover. Sean sees a private psychiatrist who has diagnosed him with generalised anxiety disorder (GAD). He wants to take the medications prescribed but he fears the drowsiness that comes with it. He was scheduled for counselling sessions with a psychologist but cannot attend any of them due to his work schedule. After all, his performance as a junior doctor is already not great, and he cannot afford to take any more time off work. Furthermore, he cannot possibly tell anyone at work about his struggles. Sean thinks for sure that he will be blacklisted if the senior doctors knew about his anxiety issues. He fears that his career will be ruined forever if this ever gets out.

Many junior doctors have a great deal of anxiety at work, even if they do not suffer from GAD. The stress of performing at 110% all the time despite feeling inadequate, the inconsistency of work schedules, and the very real possibility of some life-threatening event happening at any moment are just some of the many reasons why we might struggle with anxiety. Furthermore, our anxieties can arise from other things other than daily work issues: worries about career progression, finding a life partner, strained relationships with our families, financial struggles all cause us to have a basal level of anxiety that we carry around with us as baggage. In addition to all of this, imposter syndrome is a well-documented phenomenon amongst medical professionals, and we all harbour this fear that we will be found out to be incapable, incompetent, and undeserving of this "doctor" title which we hold.

In His sovereignty, God recognises that we frail human beings always struggle with anxiety. Hence, He gives us a host of verses throughout His Word to encourage us. The psalmist in Psalm 94:19 declares: "When anxiety was great within me, your consolation brought me joy". Jesus preaches in Matthew 6:33–34: "But seek first his kingdom and his righteousness, and all these things will be given to you as well. Therefore do not worry about tomorrow, for tomorrow will worry about itself. Each day has enough trouble of its own". Peter writes in 1 Peter 5:6–7: "Humble yourselves, therefore, under God's mighty hand, that he may lift you up in due time. Cast all your anxiety on him because he cares for you."

These are all reassurances that God knows that we are scared, and yet encourages us through His Word not to be. In this chapter, let us focus on what Paul writes to the Philippian church on the topic of anxiety, and his instructions on how we can fight it.

Anxious for Nothing

Paul's entire theme of writing to the Philippians was this: To continue to remain faithful to the Lord and to be united. With this backdrop, he writes to the church to rejoice and gave all of us readers a template in dealing with our anxiety. In Philippians 4:4–7, he breaks down how we are to approach our anxiety in several key ways. Philippians 4:4–7 says:

4 Rejoice in the Lord always. I will say it again: Rejoice! 5 Let your gentleness be evident to all. The Lord is near. 6 Do not be anxious about anything, but in every situation, by prayer and petition, with thanksgiving, present your requests to God. 7 And the peace of God, which transcends all understanding, will guard your hearts and your minds in Christ Jesus.

Rejoice in the Lord Always

The first thing that Paul tells the Philippian people to do is rejoice. He says it as a command and a verb. It is therefore not to be understood as a fleeting emotion or a "just be happy" remark. Furthermore, the Church of Jesus Christ was to actively rejoice and celebrate *in the Lord*. This meant that Paul is telling them to rejoice in His Character, His promises, what He has done for His Church, and His continued presence with us.

Therefore, the joy that we are commanded to have is not because of the absence of problems, but rather the acknowledgement of our sovereign and almighty God. Imagine a young child who is scared in a dark room and is crying out in fear. Suddenly, his father appears and holds his hand and says, "Don't worry son, I am here with you." This child will immediately feel better; he might even stop crying. He is not less afraid of the dark but is now much more reassured because of the presence of his father who he knows will provide safety, security, and a way out of the dark room.

We anxious Christians are like this young child, crippled and scared because of the many worries that besiege us from all sides. God does not always swoop down and destroy the things we fear. But He has provided Himself (the Holy Spirit) to be with us. As Paul clearly states: "the Lord is near" (verse 5). God has literally called Himself Immanuel, meaning "God with us" (Isaiah 7:14).

He has also given His Living Word (the Bible) to us, with it giving us His promises of salvation and revealing to us His character. The person of Jesus is a testament to us that God has already came down to save us at maximum cost: His own life. It is through this lens that Paul commands us to rejoice in the face of our anxieties.

Gentleness

Paul then proceeds to tell the Philippian church that they should "let their gentleness be evident to all". This is more than likely related to Galatians 5:22-23, where Paul encourages the Galatian people to have the fruit of the spirit.

"But the fruit of the Spirit is love, joy, peace, patience, kindness, goodness, faithfulness, gentleness, self-control; against such things there is no law."

Most of us will not use the abovementioned words to describe ourselves when we are anxious, whether at work or otherwise. Much of the time, we find ourselves reacting to others with rudeness, vindictiveness, or even anger when we are anxious and worried about all our responsibilities. We raise our voice when nurses call us, adding to our rapidly growing to do list. We roll our eyes when patients' family members ask us to give bedside updates on top of all the work we need to do. We brush aside and refuse to help our juniors because we already have too many things to worry about. Honestly speaking, all these responses are not surprising and frankly quite understandable. But God calls us to stand apart and commands us to be gentle. Not only that, but to let our gentleness be evident to all those around us.

Max Lucado writes in his book *Anxious for Nothing*:

"The Greek word translated here as gentleness (epiekes) describes a temperament that is seasoned and mature. It envisions an attitude that is fitting to the occasion, level-headed and tempered. The gentle reaction is one of steadiness, even-handedness, fairness. It looks humanely and reasonably at the facts of a case. Its opposite would be an overreaction or a sense of panic."

Prayer, Petition, and Thanksgiving

Again, in verse 6, Paul commands us not to be anxious. Most times, when people tell us "Stop being anxious" or "Don't worry so much", it tends to have little to no effect in helping to ease the tension. However, Paul in this case is directing us to take alternative actions. Instead of being anxious, we are commanded to present our requests to God through prayer and petition! This is a very important step to take as it focuses our thoughts on our one and only hope: God. In our great need and anxiety, we are called by the Bible to take action by going on our knees in prayer. This is important because instead of fretting about our own ability to take on the issues that we face, we turn our attention and focus on God, who is all powerful and all knowing. In doing this, we can start to right-size our problems in relation to God. True, our problems might be big. But because God is so much bigger, so mighty and so powerful, our fears naturally start to look small in comparison. We are called to remember that the God who created the world and who now dwells in us is the provider and the deliverer of His people and can certainly bring us through our problems.

But it does not stop there. We are also to partake in thanksgiving. It seems almost counterintuitive to say this here, since we usually have nothing to thank God for when we are caught in the midst of our fears. However, thanksgiving is a very formative and important exercise. As Christians, there are likely to have been times that we have seen God's goodness over our lives, whether through direct provision or through other individuals. Furthermore, our current circumstances are sure to provide examples of God's goodness: simple daily blessings such as "I have enough food on the table everyday" or "I have my family supporting me". Sometimes, we can even see how blessed we are to have the intellectual and physical capability to practise medicine.

Thanksgiving can and should bring our eyes to our own past experiences and recognise when God has been there and blessed us. In a sense, when we give thanks to God for the many things we have taken for granted, our past testifies to our present that God is good, and we need not worry.

Peace of God

The 'Peace of God' is mentioned twice in close proximity in this particular passage in Philippians, both in verse 7 and 9.

Paul first talks about the peace of God that transcends all understanding. This peace transcends all understanding because it is not some inner peace that we can manufacture through mindfulness and yoga. We cannot will ourselves to have this peace, nor necessarily even grasp it. It transcends understanding because this peace is granted despite the situations that we might be facing. Paul in uniquely qualified to say this because he himself faced trials of many kinds that are way more distressing than those that we face in the medical field. But he was able to write this passage because he knew and lived with this peace even though he was put in jail multiple times, beaten, chased out of places, and even shipwrecked. This does not mean he did not experience fear or frustration in those scenarios. But this did mean that he stuck to God's call throughout without succumbing to despair.

Furthermore, this peace is not a momentary "feel good" emotion that comes in short acting doses. The Bible tells us that the peace of God will guard our hearts against the anxiety that might assault us at random times of the day, and this peace will guard our minds against the worries and thoughts that flood in at the slightest whim. It is critical also to recognise that Paul writes that the peace of God will guard our hearts *in Christ Jesus*. This means that it is not through our own discipline or some method that we get this peace. We cannot obtain it through any power, except by the recognition that Jesus Christ is the Lord of our lives. We must remain in Jesus if we are to have this peace, seeing as Jesus is the main vine and we are the branches (John 15).

Changing the way we think and live

Paul continues this passage by writing in Philippians 4:8–9:

8 Finally, brothers and sisters, whatever is true, whatever is noble, whatever is right, whatever is pure, whatever is lovely, whatever is admirable—if anything is excellent or praiseworthy—think about such things. 9 Whatever you have learned or received or heard from me, or seen in me—put it into practice. And the God of peace will be with you.

He makes a final appeal to his readers to think about whatever is true, noble, right, pure, lovely, admirable, excellent, or praiseworthy. Besides prayer, petition, and thanksgiving, he wants them to direct their thoughts away from our worries and anxieties, and to cast them on things that are edifying and true. We know that he has pastored and mentored the Philippian church as a whole. Hence he directs them to 'put into practice' or to live out the example that was set for them in how to live out their lives as living sacrifices. In essence, Paul is saying to imitate him as he imitates Christ (1 Corinthians 11:1). He asserts therefore that if we daily change the way we think and the way we act and direct both our thoughts and actions towards Christ, that peace of God will continue to be with us throughout the tough situations.

Living out our faith

This is fine in theory but is insanely hard to do practically. It takes a superhuman level of discipline to remind yourself in the moment of anxiety that we are to direct our thoughts towards godly things instead of the things that we fear most.

On one hand, this is why it is important to consistently remain in God's Word. To pray daily and to have the habit of turning to Him whenever we fumble. As doctors, we tend to fall back onto our intellect, what we learnt in medical school, or the standard operating procedures in the hospital. Yet in the moments of chaos, we often forget to turn to God, the greatest healer we have ever known. All of us know that it takes daily practice of medicine to remain current and sharp, so we can diagnose and treat a disease with speed and accuracy. It is not enough to know the theory and then expect to react appropriately in a clinical emergency when we do not face the issues on a consistent basis. The same goes for the control of our thoughts and our actions. We will not readily turn our minds towards godly things if we do not already consistently do it. Our Bible reading, quiet times of prayer, and walking with other Christians are spiritual disciplines of grace, given by God as daily practice for the times that chaos hits.

Perhaps more importantly though, we need to be around people who will remind us to turn our thoughts to God. Even the best, most solid Christians in the world need help. We all need reminders because we are all frail and imperfect, bound to stumble and incapable of doing this on our own. Part of God's grace is that He knows all this. He knows that we are incapable of doing this alone and so He provides the Church to surround us. Living out our faith involves being accountable with other brothers and sisters in Christ. In the above passage, Paul was not telling individual Christians to sort themselves out. He was encouraging the entire church of Philippi to collectively do these things. The Bible calls us to encourage one another, to walk with each other, and to bear one another's burdens.

Being at work does not exempt us from this call. If we are not doing well, we need to seek accountability groups and form Christian relationships that enable us to remind each other of the call to change the way we think and live. If we are doing well, we open our eyes, ears, and hearts to spot others who need that help. We then play the role of being a vessel of God's blessing to others, to point them to Christ.

Discussion questions:

1. Share a time when you felt overwhelmed by anxiety or stress in your work or personal life. In what ways can you relate to Sean's experience of anxiety at work?

2. How does the act of presenting requests to God through prayer, petition, and thanksgiving help in dealing with anxiety?

3. How does directing your thoughts toward godly things contribute to experiencing the peace of God?

4. Discuss the practical challenges of consistently turning your thoughts toward God in the midst of anxiety. How can spiritual disciplines like daily Bible reading and prayer help in this regard?

5. How can Christian relationships and accountability groups support individuals facing stress and anxiety? How can we actively encourage and support our colleagues or friends who may be struggling with anxiety at work or in their personal lives?

DEPRESSION

Depression rates amongst junior doctors are significantly higher than in the general population[7]. We as Christian doctors are not spared from this affliction. Exacerbating factors include long working hours, sleep deprivation, fears of inadequacy, workplace bullying, and so on. None of these things mentioned above are exactly surprising. However, we must recognise that it does affect junior doctors, and often can have devastating consequences. Furthermore, for some reason, it is especially hard for doctors to admit that we are struggling with depression, much less start to seek help for it. It is well documented in literature that physicians tend to remain silent about their struggles with mental health and

---

[7] Tong SC, Tin AS, Tan DM, Lim JF. The health-related quality of life of junior doctors. Annals of the Academy of Medicine-Singapore. 2012 Oct 1;41(10):444.

even self-mediate in an attempt to continue functioning at work[8].

There is no easy or neat way to address issues like this. As in clinical medicine, there is no one-size-fits-all solution that we can tell any junior doctor to "cure" their depression. The journey of recovery is often much more complex and may involve a lot of grappling with deep rooted traumas, idols, and sins. However, we can rest in the knowledge that the Holy Spirit intercedes for us even when we don't know how to pray, and that God works for the good of all who love Him, and who has been called according to His purpose (Romans 8:26–28).

It is okay to be depressed

Christians are not immune to depression, and having faith in Jesus does not preclude us from experiencing mental health crises. Sometimes, we as doctors perhaps recognise that we are depressed yet have decided not to seek help. We might even have found effective ways to cover this up, and even to excel at our work while being clinically depressed. The stigma and fear that we might harbour about other people finding out about our mental health struggles may lead us keep it perpetually under wraps, which further

---

[8] Outhoff K. Depression in doctors: A bitter pill to swallow. South African Family Practice. 2019 Jun 7.

cements the problem. Perhaps the first step to addressing all of this then, is the acceptance that we are not any less if we suffer from depression.

Depression in the Bible

Mental illness is actually also featured in the stories of the Bible. Though the writers do not often interpret them in the way that modern clinicians would, they are nonetheless true and can be examined to see that people in those stories likely had what modern individuals would call "mental illnesses". One key example of depression is who God declared a man 'after [His] own heart'. King David wrote a large portion of the Psalms, and in those songs, he describes his prayers, emotions, and actions in many parts of his life. We can see from his own descriptions that he likely suffered from major depressive disorder at multiple points in his life (for a more detailed explanation, check out *Grace for the Afflicted* by Matthew S Stanford), though that diagnosis did not existed at the time.

Despite this, David was instrumental in God's plans for His people Israel. He was the first king to unite all of Israel and reigned in Israel's golden age. Furthermore, the action of writing his depression into the psalms (e.g., Psalm 6, 42, 43) meant that they could act as songs or literature for God's people to use for centuries to relate their own sadness and grief to God. The Bible does not censor nor hide the depression that David felt, but instead puts all the raw emotions on display. God's living Word therefore includes vivid accounts of David's depression. God was able to work in David and through him even in his dark times.

Like David, we are not called to censor our depression and struggle. We must understand that a biblical view of mental illness is to be unashamed of said mental illness. We are called to model after David and cry out to God in prayer and in song, perhaps even use our experiences to later help others who face the same issues, not to hide it and bury it so no one will know.

An excellent resource for Christians struggling with depression is John Piper's book *When the Darkness will not Lift*. He gives an example of how John Newton (writer of the song 'Amazing Grace') reached out to a severely depressed fellow pastor: William Cowper. Cowper would struggle his entire life with depression and suicidality, but in his depression he wrote many beautiful hymns still sung today. John Piper writes: "*without his struggles he probably would not have written 'There is a Fountain Filled with Blood' and brought hope to thousands of sinners who fear they have sinned their lives away... And he would not have written 'God Moves in a Mysterious Way' and by it helped me and many others through a hundred thickets of discouragement.*"

We, like King David and William Cowper, can continue to be vessels of God's blessing, no matter what our emotions are. As long as we are willing to live lives that are dedicated to Him, we should not feel shame about the struggles we have with depression. You can and must allow God to work through you to do productive and valuable things for Christ and your fellow brothers and sisters in healthcare. And perhaps one of the foremost steps will be to seek help and support to stabilise yourself, casting aside shame and fear that comes with being a doctor with a mental health struggle. To illustrate this point, let us examine the depressive episode of Elijah, one of our "heroes of the faith".

The Prophet Elijah: In the depth of depression and burnout, God Provides

The Old Testament Prophet Elijah is remembered as one of the great prophets of God, who stood against the prophets of the pagan god Baal. Those who know Bible stories about Elijah might remember him as the prophet who challenged the Baal prophets to a "duel" in order to see which of their Gods was more powerful. In 1 Kings 18:16–40, Elijah asked them to call on Baal to light the fire on the altar for them. They failed miserably and Elijah proceeded to show them the power of the God of Israel. The result was spectacular, as God provided a fire so strong that it consumed the sacrifice on the altar, the wood, the stone, and even the water in the surrounding trench. He had a massive victory that day, and he showed the Baal prophets and all of Israel that the one true God was the one to be worshipped. He even managed to convince the people watching. In verse 39, the Bible records that *"when all the people saw this, they fell prostrate and cried, 'the Lord – He is God! The Lord – He is God!'"*. This was a major victory for Elijah, a prophet of God trying to turn his people back to Him.

What we tend to forget (or plainly not know) is that almost immediately after, Elijah was faced with persecution and fell into depression. In 1 Kings 19:1–21, Jezebel (the pagan queen of Israel and wife to King Ahab) made a death threat to Elijah for what he did to the Baal prophets. Elijah ran for his life and hid. He then experienced some of the lowest moods recorded in the Bible. He struggled so hard because he felt rejected and that his life's work was for nothing. He lamented to God that though he has been zealous, the Israelites have not responded in kind and have rejected him and killed other prophets of God (verse 10). He was so upset that he became suicidal, praying to God that he might die. In verse 4, Elijah says "I've had enough, Lord. Take my life, I am no better than my ancestors". This is shocking because he does not just feel like dying, but actively asks God to kill him because he has had enough.

We are sometimes like Elijah

As junior doctors, we sometimes find our lives paralleled by Elijah's story in 1 Kings 19. Being a doctor is often thought of as glamourous and is rightfully a source of pride. We slog through five to seven years of university and win a great victory by passing our exams and becoming qualified as a doctor. Yet, it does not take long after graduation for things to become a depressive, hard slog. Elijah's depression similarly came after he defeated and killed the prophets of Baal. He spent his life serving God and displayed God's awesome power to Israel and to the Baal prophets. Like graduating from medical school, this too was a huge effort and a great victory for Elijah.

However, this victory of Elijah's was not only not rewarded, but he was given a death threat and was forced into hiding, living in fear and dread daily. In stark contrast to the bravery he displayed when facing the 450 Baal prophets the chapter before, Elijah's courage quickly melted away in the face of the queen's threat. Furthermore, he felt like all that he accomplished had been for nothing. He won a great victory and even managed to convince some of the Israelites present at the miracle to worship God again. But this resulted in the death threat and rejection again by the people of Israel as a whole. He must have felt frustrated and helpless, like nothing he could do would overcome the evil ways of Israel.

Similarly, we junior doctors often feel overwhelmed and threatened by the immense workload and sometimes nasty workplace culture. Though we may not experience death threats, we harbour many fears of what might happen at work, making mistakes, or not performing up to par. Furthermore, we are often plagued by frustrations at the inadequacies of the system, unfairness of the workplace we find ourselves in, and recalcitrant patients. We might also feel that we make no difference no matter how much effort we put in as junior doctors.

The manifestation of our frustration and anxiety is therefore similarly relatable to the prophet Elijah. We, like him, experience a sense of meaninglessness, disappointment, and often feel burnt out. Some of us even slip into depression, facing anhedonia, loss of motivation, and even suicidal ideation.

God provides

The good news is God knows our frustration and He hears our cries. His guidance of Elijah stands as a model of how we can start to approach God in the times we feel depressed. After his suicidal outburst, Elijah falls asleep in the shade of a broom tree (v5). God then sends an angel who touched Elijah and gave him bread and water to eat. He ate and drank and fell asleep again, only to be woken up a second time by the angel (v7) before being directed to Horeb, the mountain of God (v8). Elijah then travels to Horeb and to speak to God.

God provides physical rest

First of all, God calls us to physical rest. God sent an angel with bread and water to feed Elijah (v5). He provided a shaded spot (the broom tree) for Elijah to rest, and later directed him to Horeb, the mountain of God (v8). Before letting him go, the angel of the Lord interestingly insisted a second time that Elijah should eat and drink, because if he did not, the journey would be too much for him.

This is significant because before any form of spiritual encounter, the story first focuses on the physical nourishment of Elijah. Physical rest is a deeply biblical concept, and the Judaeo-Christian understanding of body-mind-spirit is that they are deeply connected (instead of separate entities, which is more of a Greek/western understanding). Therefore, the writers of 1 Kings thought it important enough include these details in the text. In the same way, physical rest is not something we should take lightly or neglect. In Psalm 23:1–3 David writes:

The Lord is my shepherd, I lack nothing. He makes me lie down in green pastures, he leads me beside quiet waters, he refreshes my soul.

Scripture clearly helps us to recognise that physical rest and sustenance is a provision of the Lord. That is why David writes about God making him lie down, leading him, and refreshing his soul. Just as Elijah went to Horeb after resting, physical rest should lead us into a place of seeking God. Many of us think that physical rest (sleeping, relaxing, and entertainment) is separate from spiritual rejuvenation (healing of our souls, connecting with God, or worship). However, the true biblical idea of rest encompasses both the physical and spiritual.

God provides spiritual rest

a) God draws us into his presence

The presence of God is a powerful thing. It reminds us of His might and glory, and makes all else on Earth fade away. Elijah needed to follow God's leading to stand on the mountain, so as to encounter God's presence (v11). Then a powerful wind came, followed by an earthquake, followed by a fire. However, God was not to be found in any of these dramatic ways. Instead, He came in a gentle whisper ("a still small voice") to speak to Elijah. This shows us that the voice of God may not be loud or dramatic, and often we need to be attentive and still before Him in order to hear it.

To be clear, God can appear in dramatic ways and often did so in the Bible (e.g., a pillar of fire in Exodus). But in this case,

He chose to whisper, and Elijah heard Him and went out of the cave.

If we are feeling down, perhaps a good question to ask ourselves then is: how have we felt God's presence before? Do we feel His presence now? If He seems to be completely absent from our lives at the moment, could it be because our hearts are so full of noise that we fail to hear His still small voice? Perhaps we need to say to ourselves: "be still my anxious heart", take a step back and like Elijah, wait quietly in the cave and listen attentively for His presence.

b) God reminds us of his purpose for us (v14-16)

Elijah twice voices his frustration that Israel had not turned back to God even after all that he did, as if all that he did counted for nothing (v10, v14). God replies him, but does not answer Elijah directly. Instead, He gives Elijah a list of instructions: go to Damascus, anoint Hazael, anoint Jehu, anoint Elisha (v15–16). With this, Elijah regained his strength and departed to do as he was told. We don't get an explanation as to how and why Elijah recovered. We do not even get a clear idea of how long Elijah spent on the mountain communicating with God and recovering. Perhaps this is left ambiguous on purpose because those particular details are not the point. The point is that Elijah's conversation with God led him to new purpose.

Sometimes, it is hard to see God's purpose in our lives, especially when what we do seems to count for nothing. But God does have a purpose for each of us in His Kingdom. It may be a greatly revered task; it may be a humble purpose. We do not always know it, but we can be sure that it will be exactly right for us. Our job is not to scheme and plan our lives for the greatest potential, but to spend our days living faithfully under God's will and communing with Him. When He has a task for us, He will send us. Then, we need to have the humility to obey.

Though being a doctor is traditionally thought of as glamourous, all of us know that the mundane and sometimes irksome jobs of junior doctors are far from that. It is liberating however to see that all we do is a direct service to God's Kingdom and to love His children. This is a blessing that others in different career paths might not always enjoy. We get to participate in a ministry unto His people in the worst parts of their lives (when they are sick), and we get the privilege of being a vessel of His tangible blessing. Remembering that purpose daily should point our hearts to gratitude and to God Himself.

c) God assures us of his control over creation (v17–18)

Finally, in response to Elijah's complaint that "nothing has changed", God reveals to Elijah His plans to exert justice on Israel and to save a remnant of 7000 for himself (v17–18).

At this point, Elijah would not know what exactly God is doing with those 7000 people. However, what is clear is that God is in control, even when things seem completely out of hand.

Perhaps this teaches us that it is right to be frustrated at a flawed or unjust system. We are not called to be blind and mute cogs in the system. However, we need to remember that God is in control. He enacts His perfect will through imperfect things (such as ourselves) and will always prevail. Our job is to know that He is in charge and that He is working for the good of those who love Him (Romans 8:28).

God provides co-workers to share the load.

Elijah had previously proudly and bravely proclaimed that he alone stood up for God (1 Kings 18:22). But in chapter 19, that sense of pride had turned to self-pity, and he felt alone in this fight (v10). Interestingly, Elijah at this point seems to have forgotten about the 100 prophets who were protected by Obadiah just one chapter before (1 Kings 18:4,13). But more importantly, this particular passage is immediately followed up by the call of Elisha, who will eventually become Elijah's protégé and bring spiritual discernment and the Lord's further judgement to Israel. It is not a coincidence Elijah's bout of depression is immediately followed by the call of Elisha.

From this point on, God provided Elijah with a co-worker in ministry, and one who will eventually take over after Elijah was taken from Earth. This also stands as one of God's answers to Elijah's depression: that God provides him a co-worker so that he might not be alone. This is a deep idea that is consistent with the New Testament where the disciples are never working alone but always in community. Furthermore, the way that the Christian Church has functioned since her inception shows that none of us are to be labouring alone for God. Yes, we are sometimes persecuted, and we are often hard-pressed from every side, but having a community of co-labourers in the Lord is an important prophylaxis against depression and burnout.

This is why it is so important not to neglect our communities even when we get busy. Many of us stop meeting up with accountability groups (e.g., cell, Bible study groups) and might find ourselves consistently missing church. This is understandable and none of us should condemn each other for having done that due to tiredness or lack of time. However, we need to commit to look out for one other and allow others to look out for us. We need the accountability of close Christian brothers and sisters in Christ or mentors to tell us what we need to hear and to cover our blind spots. Like the previous chapter on anxiety, we need to approach those we trust and ask them to journey alongside us on the road to recovery. If necessary, we must put aside our pride and fears of career delay and seek professional help.

As we toil, we are to share the load with our co-workers in Christ, and together look to Jesus who promises that His yoke is easy, and His burden is light. Community is the setting which we have been created to function, and without it we tend to crumble.

We are not alone

This depression we so often see in our medical community is nothing new. There is precedent in Scripture and God gracefully provides us with some answers. If even the great Prophet Elijah or the great King David can become depressed, burnt out, and even suicidal, there is no shame nor surprise that we ordinary folk are equally vulnerable. The Bible does not avoid nor sugar-coat depression. Instead, it repeatedly insists on the greater promise that God will provide. He will provide physical rest, He will provide spiritual rest, and He will provide co-workers to share the load. But most of all, He has provided a Saviour that has redeemed our work and will one day come again to make all things new and perfect. Through the storms of life, we have this sure and steadfast anchor of our soul (Hebrews 6:19).

Discussion Questions:

1. In what ways might the expectations and pressures in the medical profession contribute to mental health struggles, and how can we combat this in our personal lives?

2. Why do you think the Bible openly discusses the emotional and mental challenges of its prominent figures, such as David and Elijah?

3. Why do you think it's challenging for individuals, particularly doctors, to admit and seek help for depression? How can the church community contribute to a more accepting environment?

4. Discuss Elijah's emotional journey from a great victory to deep depression. What spiritual and practical lessons can we draw from God's response to Elijah's depression?

5. How does God redefine Elijah's purpose during his time of despair? How can understanding our purpose in God's Kingdom impact our perspective during challenging times?

6. Discuss the importance of community and co-workers in combating depression and burnout. How can we encourage a supportive community in our workplaces and churches?

EPILOGUE: HOPE IN THE LORD

Our lives are a tapestry woven with threads of challenges and triumphs, moments of doubt and unwavering faith. The medical field we find ourselves in often gives us immense pressure. It is therefore crucial to hold on to our hope in Christ like an anchor in the storm.

The journey of a junior doctor is not an easy one, but it is a calling filled with purpose and meaning. It is a ministry of healing and compassion, where our hands become instruments of God's grace. In the midst of long hours and difficult decisions, may we always remember that we are not alone. God walks beside us, guiding our steps and renewing our spirits. Our fellow Christians are in the trenches with us, fighting alongside and encouraging us.

Let us continue to lift each other up in prayer and support. And may we always find solace in the words of Isaiah 40:31,

"but those who hope in the Lord

will renew their strength.

They will soar on wings like eagles;

they will run and not grow weary,

they will walk and not be faint."

May God bless you abundantly in your journey as a Christian doctor, and may your life and the work of your hands be a shining testament to His love and grace.

www.ingramcontent.com/pod-product-compliance
Lightning Source LLC
LaVergne TN
LVHW021237080526
838199LV00088B/4548